Essential Articles in Colorectal Surgery

AF166647

Dorin Colibaseanu
Michelle DeLeon · Amit Merchea
Luca Stocchi

Essential Articles in Colorectal Surgery

Four Colleagues Discuss
the Evidence and Their
Experience

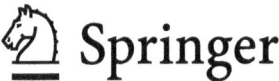 Springer

Dorin Colibaseanu
Division of Colorectal Surgery
Mayo Clinic Florida
Jacksonville, FL, USA

Michelle DeLeon
Division of Colorectal Surgery
Mayo Clinic Florida
Jacksonville, FL, USA

Amit Merchea
Division of Colorectal Surgery
Mayo Clinic Florida
Jacksonville, FL, USA

Luca Stocchi
Division of Colorectal Surgery
Mayo Clinic Florida
Jacksonville, FL, USA

ISBN 978-3-031-77744-8   ISBN 978-3-031-77745-5   (eBook)
https://doi.org/10.1007/978-3-031-77745-5

© The Editor(s) (if applicable) and The Author(s), under exclusive license to
Springer Nature Switzerland AG 2025, Corrected Publication 2025

This work is subject to copyright. All rights are solely and exclusively licensed by
the Publisher, whether the whole or part of the material is concerned, specifically
the rights of translation, reprinting, reuse of illustrations, recitation, broadcasting,
reproduction on microfilms or in any other physical way, and transmission or
information storage and retrieval, electronic adaptation, computer software, or by
similar or dissimilar methodology now known or hereafter developed.
The use of general descriptive names, registered names, trademarks, service
marks, etc. in this publication does not imply, even in the absence of a specific
statement, that such names are exempt from the relevant protective laws and
regulations and therefore free for general use.
The publisher, the authors and the editors are safe to assume that the advice and
information in this book are believed to be true and accurate at the date of
publication. Neither the publisher nor the authors or the editors give a warranty,
expressed or implied, with respect to the material contained herein or for any
errors or omissions that may have been made. The publisher remains neutral with
regard to jurisdictional claims in published maps and institutional affiliations.

This Springer imprint is published by the registered company Springer Nature
Switzerland AG
The registered company address is: Gewerbestrasse 11, 6330 Cham, Switzerland

If disposing of this product, please recycle the paper.

Foreword

There has been a tremendous evolution in the surgical care of patients with diseases of the colon, rectum, and anus over the last one hundred years. This evolution has been driven by many factors, including improved understanding of disease, surgical training, specialization, and research. Due to the important work of academic surgeons, practice in the modern era is guided by a foundation of scientific evidence that can significantly improve the quality-of-care patients receive. Critical analysis and sometimes passionate debate of data published in surgical journals is a common academic exercise to determine if a study's findings meet a sufficient standard to change practice. These important discussions of published data occur in conference rooms, lecture halls, and at local, regional, national, and international meetings. This book *Essential Articles in Colorectal Surgery* takes this process of critical analysis among surgeons out of lecture halls and academic meetings and puts it on the written page.

The authors are to be congratulated for the unique design of this book. Drawing on landmark peer-reviewed studies, the authors have curated a resource that allows the reader to appreciate how four surgeons, who work together, interpret and put into practice the findings of 40 highly relevant papers in the specialty of colon and rectal surgery. The findings of these carefully selected papers have been summarized and are then discussed between the four surgeons, allowing the reader to appreciate how each surgeon understands the data and its relevance to their day-to-day practice.

I found this book highly educational, thoughtfully drafted, and comprehensive across the diverse practice of colon and rectal surgery. More than just a repository of published data, this work emphasizes the dynamic nature of how this data is interpreted and then put into practice. It challenges us to consider not only what we know but also how we know it and how we can continue to improve the rigor and relevance of the studies that guide us.

For clinicians, researchers, and students alike, this book is a reminder of the responsibility we all bear in medicine, which is to seek truth, to question assumptions, and to apply knowledge in ways that are ethical and effective. Published research often makes us ask more questions that need answers, and this book aims to inspire the pursuit of new knowledge in the rapidly changing field of colon and rectal surgery.

Chair, Division of Colorectal Surgery   Eric J. Dozois, MD
Mayo Clinic Rochester MN
USA

Contents

The original version of the book has been revised. A correction to this book
can be found at https://doi.org/10.1007/978-3-031-77745-5_41

Are Resection Margins Important in Crohn's Disease?

Truong A, Chough J, Zaghiyan KN, Fleshner PR. Risk factors for microscopic disease positivity at ileocolic resection margins for Crohn's disease. Surg Technol Int. 2024;44:99–104.

Abstract

Introduction: Interest in microscopic margin positivity during surgical resection for medically refractory Crohn's disease has been renewed by multiple recent studies showing an association between microscopic margin positivity with disease recurrence. Our aim was to determine the risk factors for microscopic margin disease positivity following ileocolic resection (ICR).

Materials and Methods: A prospectively maintained database of patients with Crohn's disease undergoing ICR at a tertiary-referral center was queried. Margin positivity was defined as the presence of cryptitis, erosion, transmural inflammation with lymphoid aggregates, or architectural distortion at either ileal (proximal) or colonic (distal) margins.

Results: Among 584 patients, 97 patients had a positive microscopic margin (17%), of which 46% had a positive proximal margin, 17% had a positive distal margin, and 13% had both positive and distal margins. Using multivariable logistic regression analysis, index ICR was associated with less odds of positive margin (odds ratio [OR] 0.46, 95% confidence interval [CI] 0.24–0.89,

© The Author(s), under exclusive license to Springer Nature Switzerland AG 2025
D. Colibaseanu et al., *Essential Articles in Colorectal Surgery*,
https://doi.org/10.1007/978-3-031-77745-5_1

$p = 0.02$), and granuloma presence was associated with increased odds (OR 2.26, 95% CI 1.23–4.21, $p = 0.01$).

Conclusion: We found that repeat ileocolic resection and granuloma presence were predictors of microscopic margin disease.

DC

This is a single institution study of 584 patients addressing the question of what risk factors are associated with a positive microscopic margin after surgery for Crohn's disease (CD). This is a very important question to answer, as microscopically positive margins are associated with recurrence of disease [1] and, in some of these recurrences, repeated need for surgery. The macroscopic appearance of a disease-free margin does not always correlate with the microscopic analysis [1, 2]. This is not at all a new concern, and it has been attempted to be answered in the past; some associations were drawn, but the studies were often small and not necessarily done at high-volume IBD centers [3]. Other studies have found that smoking and even the number of cigarettes smoked per day had an association with recurrence but also found that interestingly enough, longer macroscopically disease-free resected segments and granuloma presence were not associated with higher recurrence rates [4].

Decades later, we know that microscopically positive margins are associated with recurrence of CD at the anastomosis, but what can we do to minimize this risk? This study found that ileocecal resections have a higher risk of microscopically positive margins as did the presence of granulomas. The three questions that this brings forth are whether frozen section should be routinely employed, begging the following question, which is how aggressively we should chase "negative margins," in patients who will likely have to contemplate in the future additional bowel resections. The third question that this brings up is in which patients post resection should we pursue aggressive medical treatment, and will this aggressive treatment reduce the risk of clinical relapse which can occur in as much as half of the patients undergoing surgery [5].

References

1. Kelm M, Benatzky C, Buck V, et al. Positive resection margins in Crohn's disease are a relevant risk factor for postoperative disease recurrence. Sci Rep. 2024;14:10823. https://doi.org/10.1038/s41598-024-61697.
2. Yzet C, Ruault C, Brazier F, et al. Positive margins and plexitis increase the risk of recurrence after ileocecal resection: a systematic review and meta-analysis. Dig Liver Dis. 2023;55(12):1611–20.
3. Kotanagi H, Kramer K, Fazio VW, Petras RE. Do microscopic abnormalities at resection margins correlate with increased anastomotic recurrence in Crohn's disease? Retrospective analysis of 100 cases. Dis Colon Rectum. 1991;34(10):909–16.
4. van Hogezand RA, Bemelman WA. Management of recurrent Crohn's disease. Neth J Med. 1998;53(6):S32–8.
5. Hammoudi N, Cazals-Hatem D, Auzolle C, et al. Association between microscopic lesions at ileal resection margin and recurrence after surgery in patients with Crohn's disease. Clin Gastroenterol Hepatol. 2020;18(1):141–149.e2.

Discussion

MD

I have not seen the studies looking at increased risk of recurrence with microscopic positivity. Historically, I know we are always taught that we really just go to gross margins. So, this was interesting to see with regard to risk factors for microscopic positivity. I think we would be interested to see in the study if those patients with positive microscopic margins ended up having increased recurrence rates. I know this paper was really looking at risk factors for determining positivity. Are you guys familiar with that data? Looking at the microscopic disease?

LS

I have read some studies, and they are very heterogeneous. Among others, Bruce Wolff at Mayo Clinic in the 1980s looked into that association. At some point, there was even the impetus to have frozen sections to ensure the absence of microscopic disease before anastomosis. Ultimately, all these studies have not indicated that microscopic margins are an important individual factor predicting recurrence. The prospective randomized study by Victor Fazio in the 1990s (Fazio, Ann Surg 1996) reaffirmed the still current standard of care of aiming at grossly negative margins of resection. It compared a proximal small bowel margin of 2 cm from gross disease vs. 12 cm, and interestingly, there were some patients randomized to extended resection who still had some degree of microscopic Crohn's disease at their small bowel transection line. As far as I am concerned, the possibility of microscopic disease at the resection margins should not change our surgical management.

DC

I agree. The question that this brings up is how much effort should we put in demonstrating whether we have microscopically negative margins? And then following that, what are we going to do about it? Definitely a question worth asking, and for now, I do not know anyone who uses intraoperative frozen section to demonstrate microscopically negative margins.

MD

I agree. And I do not believe any of the gastroenterologists really look at the status of microscopic resection margins to determine whether or not they are going to place patients on medical therapy after surgery. I think what would also be interesting, now that a lot of people are doing intracorporeal anastomosis and not actually feeling the specimens is whether or not there has been a difference in positive resection margin or recurrence between robotic intracorporeal anastomosis vs. extracorporeal where it is possible to actually feel the tissue rather than just assessing the bowel by eye. I do not think that it has been looked at, but I know when I first started doing intracorporeal anastomosis, it is straightforward for the obvious, gross disease. However, for those patients with more subtle disease or who may have multifocal strictures, I am a little bit more wary, and I have extracorporealized some small bowels just to further assess it with palpation, if I am ever concerned about that.

LS

I agree. The other intervening factor in the robotic anastomosis is the anastomotic configuration, which could also become the subject of debate because most of the time we would not do isoperistaltic side-to-side anastomosis in open or laparoscopic surgery. I do not have a lot of robotic experience, but I do agree that in some cases, I felt that I could not just visually assess the presence of additional Crohn's disease somewhere else in the small bowel besides the segment which was being resected, and I decided to exteriorize because of that.

Handsewn vs. Stapled Ileocolic Anastomosis in Crohn's Disease

2

McLeod RS, Wolff BG, Ross S, Parkes R, McKenzie M, Investigators of the CAST Trial. Recurrence of Crohn's disease after ileocolic resection is not affected by anastomotic type: results of a multicenter, randomized, controlled trial. Dis Colon Rectum. 2009;52(5):919–27.

Abstract

Purpose: This study attempts to determine whether stapled side-to-side anastomosis, compared with handsewn end-to-end anastomosis, results in decreased recurrence of Crohn's disease following ileocolic resection.

Methods: Patients with Crohn's disease who underwent an ileocolic resection were randomized to side-to-side anastomosis or end-to-end anastomosis. Colonoscopy was performed at 12 months. The primary outcome was endoscopic recurrence, while the secondary outcome was symptomatic recurrence (defined as symptoms attributable to Crohn's disease and severe enough to warrant treatment, plus endoscopic disease recurrence).

Results: One hundred and thirty-nine subjects were included in the efficacy analysis. After a mean follow-up of 11.9 months, the endoscopic recurrence rate was 42.5% in the end-to-end anastomosis group, compared with 37.9% in the side-to-side anastomosis group (4.6% difference; 95% confidence interval 21.0–11.9%; $P = 0.55$). The symptomatic recurrence rate was

© The Author(s), under exclusive license to Springer Nature Switzerland AG 2025
D. Colibaseanu et al., *Essential Articles in Colorectal Surgery*, https://doi.org/10.1007/978-3-031-77745-5_2

21.9% in the end-to-end anastomosis group, compared with 22.7% in the side-to-side anastomosis group (+0.8% difference; 95% confidence interval 13.2–15.3%; P = 0.92). In multivariate logistic regression analysis, previous resections were predictive of a higher risk of both endoscopic (odds ratio 1.78; 95% confidence interval 1.06–2.90; P = 0.028) and symptomatic (odds ratio 2.0; 95% confidence interval 1.14–3.60; P = 0.0016) recurrence. Compliance with postoperative maintenance therapy was predictive of a lower risk of symptomatic recurrence (odds ratio 0.13, 95% confidence interval 0.01–0.78; P = 0.021).

Conclusion: Recurrence rates are similar whether end-to-end anastomosis or side-to-side anastomosis is performed.

LS

This is a randomized trial comparing two anastomotic techniques in the management of ileocolic resection for Crohn's disease which has defined my agnostic attitude toward this issue ever since. The Canadian and American Surgical Crohn's Disease Trial (CAST) randomized end-to-end versus side-to-side ileocolic anastomosis. This basically ended up being a comparison between handsewn versus stapled anastomosis. This trial had been designed based on the hypothesis that a wider side-to-side stapled anastomosis could be associated with a longer time to recurrence. The assumption at the time was that "a narrow anastomosis may lead to fecal stasis and increase the likelihood of recurrence of disease." The outcomes of interest were endoscopic recurrence and symptomatic recurrence. One hundred thirty-nine patients were randomized in 17 different centers. The patient enrollment in the study was stopped in 2004 due to slow accrual. After a mean follow-up of 11.9 months, there were no differences between the groups in either endoscopic or symptomatic recurrence. The anastomotic leak rates were 7% in either group. This is obviously an old trial at a time when many of the currently available medications were not available. For example, 22% and 16% of the end-to-end group and side-to-side group, respectively, were on prednisone preoperatively. Modern medical prophylaxis after surgery could be associated with improved results across the board at least in terms of endoscopic and symptomatic recurrence 1 year postoperatively. However, this study because of its design clarified the lack of benefit associated with the stapled anastomosis at least in terms of disease recurrence. This randomized trial had been planned based on some encouraging results deriving from earlier retrospective, observational studies, which are referenced in the paper. This to me confirms that observational studies should not be viewed as sufficient evidence to support the adoption of one particular anastomotic technique over another. It is interesting to note that the debate on the ideal surgical technique for ileocolic anastomosis after ileocolic resection for Crohn's disease continues to this day, almost 20 years after the accrual for this study was terminated. The European Crohn's and Colitis Organisation guidelines from 2020 continue recommending stapled rather than handsewn ileocolic anastomosis because of a decreased risk of anastomotic complications [1]. Therefore, the preference for stapled anastomosis in this case does not derive from a perceived advantage in reducing the risk of disease recurrence. At the opposite side of the spectrum, there are advocates of a handsewn anastomosis [2]. More recently, a new anastomotic technique loosely based on the surgical principles of strictureplasty was proposed by the late Dr. Toru Kono in Japan, the Kono-S anastomosis [3]. The letter "S" stands for support, which would be provided by the preservation of the mesentery close to the bowel utilized to perform the anastomosis. On the other hand, there is also a school of thought advocating wide excision of the mesentery during ileocolic resection to reduce disease recurrence [4], and the combination of wide mesenteric excision and Kono anastomosis has also been proposed [5]. A recent prospective randomized trial has suggested that Kono-S ileocolic anastomosis is associated with a reduced rate of endoscopic recurrence when compared to stapled side-to-side ileocolic anastomosis [6]. If confirmed by other similarly designed studies, this could potentially lead to a change in practice. Until then, I do not expect that any anastomotic technique is associated with a different risk of disease recurrence rate. When the small bowel proximal to a severe stricture is dilated with boggy, thickened bowel wall because of chronic obstructive symptoms, I prefer to do an end-to-end anastomosis because I am concerned that the mechanical stapler might not be effective on thickened, edematous bowel wall. On the other hand, if there is a discrepancy between a narrow diameter in the terminal ileum and a much larger ascending colon, I typically favor a side-to-side anisoperistaltic stapled anastomosis. With the advent of robotic technique and intracorporeal anastomosis, there is another anastomotic type which is gaining favor, a side-to-side isoperistaltic ileocolic anastomosis using a robotic stapler with the closure of the resulting defect using running intracorporeal sutures [7]. Advocates of the robotic approach emphasize its recovery and morbidity advantages and consider this technique safe and feasible but do not postulate any presumed benefits in reducing Crohn's disease recurrence rates.

References

1. Adamina M, Bonovas S, Raine T, Spinelli A, Warusavitarne J, Armuzzi A, Bachmann O, Bager P, Biancone L, Bokemeyer B, Bossuyt P, Burisch J, Collins P, Doherty G, El-Hussuna A, Ellul P, Fiorino G, Frei-Lanter C, Furfaro F, Gingert C, Gionchetti P, Gisbert JP, Gomollon F, González Lorenzo M, Gordon H, Hlavaty T, Juillerat P, Katsanos K, Kopylov U, Krustins E, Kucharzik T, Lytras T, Maaser C, Magro F, Marshall JK, Myrelid P, Pellino G, Rosa I, Sabino J, Savarino E, Stassen L, Torres J, Uzzan M, Vavricka S, Verstockt B, Zmora O. ECCO guidelines on therapeutics in Crohn's disease: surgical treatment. J Crohns Colitis. 2020;14(2):155–68.
2. Gajendran M, Bauer AJ, Buchholz BM, Watson AR, Koutroubakis IE, Hashash JG, Ramos-Rivers C, Shah N, Lee KK, Cruz RJ, Regueiro M, Zuckerbraun B, Schwartz M, Swoger J, Barrie A, Harrison J, Hartman DJ, Salgado J, Rivers WM, Click B, Anderson AM, Umapathy C, Babichenko D, Dunn MA, Binion DG. Ileocecal anastomosis type significantly influences long-term functional status, quality of life, and healthcare utilization in postoperative Crohn's disease patients independent of inflammation recurrence. Am J Gastroenterol. 2018;113(4):576–83.

3. Kono T, Ashida T, Ebisawa Y, Chisato N, Okamoto K, Katsuno H, Maeda K, Fujiya M, Kohgo Y, Furukawa H. A new antimesenteric functional end-to-end handsewn anastomosis: surgical prevention of anastomotic recurrence in Crohn's disease. Dis Colon Rectum. 2011;54(5):586–92.
4. Zhu Y, Qian W, Huang L, Xu Y, Guo Z, Cao L, Gong J, Coffey JC, Shen B, Li Y, Zhu W. Role of extended mesenteric excision in postoperative recurrence of Crohn's colitis: a single-center study. Clin Transl Gastroenterol. 2021;12(10):e00407.
5. Holubar SD, Gunter RL, Click BH, Achkar JP, Lightner AL, Lipman JM, Hull TL, Regueiro M, Rieder F, Steele SR. Mesenteric excision and exclusion for ileocolic Crohn's disease: feasibility and safety of an innovative, combined surgical approach with extended mesenteric excision and Kono-S anastomosis. Dis Colon Rectum. 2022;65(1):e5–13.
6. Luglio G, Rispo A, Imperatore N, Giglio MC, Amendola A, Tropeano FP, Peltrini R, Castiglione F, De Palma GD, Bucci L. Surgical prevention of anastomotic recurrence by excluding mesentery in Crohn's disease: the SuPREMe-CD Study—a randomized clinical trial. Ann Surg. 2020;272(2):210–7.
7. Calini G, Abdalla S, Abd El Aziz MA, Merchea A, Larson DW, Behm KT. Ileocolic resection for Crohn's disease: robotic intracorporeal compared to laparoscopic extracorporeal anastomosis. J Robot Surg. 2023;17(5):2157–66.

Discussion

LS

This is the study that has informed my agnostic attitude about ileocolic anastomotic technique in Crohn's disease, and I realize that saying this might not sound very exciting. I simply do not think there is any sufficient evidence to recommend one type of anastomosis over another. This becomes particularly important with the advent of robotic surgery and intracorporeal anastomosis. The side-to-side isoperistaltic stapled anastomosis is not among the anastomosis types which have been studied for the last 20 years, but my indifference to a specific technique and orientation makes me comfortable at the idea of transitioning to robotic surgery and intracorporeal anastomosis.

MD

I think this older study gives us some insight on the ongoing debate surrounding Kono-S and mesenteric sparing techniques. Decades ago, as emphasized in this paper, the focus was on end-to-end versus side-to-side approaches. Today, the conversation revolves around Kono-S, stapled, and mesenteric sparing methods. In my view, no single study provides conclusive evidence to unequivocally support any particular technique. Therefore, when considering outcomes, I firmly believe that the optimal technique is the one you are most proficient and comfortable performing.

AM

This is an area where people often describe technical aspects as critical to the outcome. But to me, Crohn's is such a situation where often the disease trumps what we may do technically. And we put, perhaps, too much importance on our own ability to do something in one manner or another surgically which we think will overcome the burden of this terrible disease.

This is why I'm indifferent as to whether it's end-to-end, side-to-side isoperistaltic or anisoperistaltic. One argument made for one technique or another is in regard to endoscopic surveillance, where it may be easier or more difficult with one over the other.

DC

I think looking at the study, it's a valiant effort. But it speaks to the difficulty of actually carrying out a study like this, 170 patients total, across multiple institutions and multiple continents. The patients are not homogeneous, and it is hard to account for even the obvious confounders. It's very hard to have a homogeneous type of population, yet it would be hard to have a bigger study to look at this question. This is the best we have, and I think that if there was a difference, it's so small that it would be hard to capture it with 178 patients. My take home is that there's no obvious difference between the two.

LS

Gastroenterologists do not seem to put a lot of emphasis on the potential differences among different anastomotic techniques in endoscopic surveillance, which is a point Amit was making and I also wondered about. However, apart from theoretical concerns, it does not seem to be a very relevant clinical issue.

MD

I do remember Bo Shen (IBD gastroenterologist) when he was at Cleveland Clinic would always say that an end-to-side, which is often done in Cleveland Clinic, is actually easier to intubate than a traditional side-to-side.

But perhaps that was just anecdotal for him.

LS

I remember he was saying that, but in reference to a comparison between those two specific anastomotic techniques. At the UPMC (University of Pittsburgh Medical Center), both gastroenterologists and surgeons favor an end-to-end handsewn anastomosis all the time because of concerns not related to demonstrable differences in disease recurrence rate, but because there would be other disadvantages that are putatively ascribed to fecal stasis and possible bacterial overgrowth when leaving a blind limb. This argument is not convincing to me. The advent of the Kono-S anastomosis has further intensified this ongoing debate which has continued for many years since the CAST study is about 20 years old.

AM

And I think the other thing you have to balance with how you do these techniques and the era in which some of these arguments were made is that the creation of these anastomoses often requires a more invasive approach, either through a mini laparotomy or periumbilical incision. And so, considering a patient population that almost inevitably will have future surgery, you're potentially prolonging their recovery, increasing the postoperative morbidity, whether it's hernia or wound infection, and even complicating the subsequent surgery.

So I think we also must consider for Crohn's patients what's your next operation. Not only in terms of planning to treat the current disease, but also in planning the conduct of the next operation, be it minimally invasive or not. Robotics has become the great equalizer in that it allows many things that we would always have to do open or feel like we had to do open; now because of the dexterity of the robotic platforms, we can do these things in a minimally invasive fashion.

The last comment I have is in regard to the Kono-S anastomosis, which has become rather popular for reasons I don't necessarily understand. The original description did not involve resecting the mesentery, yet how people practice that type of anastomosis often involves a wider resection. I think practically most of us probably just go to where the mesentery is soft and easy to ligate as opposed to right next to the bowel wall where it's thickened and inflamed or right along the origin of the feeding vessel where there is higher risk and a higher likelihood of more extensive bowel resection.

Use of TNFα Inhibitors and Surgery for Crohn's Disease

3

Cohen BL, Fleshner P, Kane SV, et al. Prospective cohort study to investigate the safety of preoperative tumor necrosis factor inhibitor exposure in patients with inflammatory bowel disease undergoing intra-abdominal surgery. Gastroenterology. 2022;163(1):204–21.

Abstract

Background and Aim: Whether preoperative treatment of inflammatory bowel disease (IBD) with tumor necrosis factor inhibitors (TNFis) increases the risk of postoperative infectious complications remains controversial. The primary aim of this study was to determine whether preoperative exposure to TNFis is an independent risk factor for postoperative infectious complications within 30 days of surgery.

Methods: We conducted a multicenter prospective observational study of patients with IBD undergoing intra-abdominal surgery across 17 sites from the Crohn's and Colitis Foundation Clinical Research Alliance. Infectious complications were categorized as surgical site infections (SSIs) or non-SSIs. Current TNFi exposure was defined as use within 12 weeks of surgery, and serum was collected for drug-level analyses. Multivariable models for occurrence of the primary outcome, any infection, or SSI were adjusted by predefined covariates (age, sex, preoperative steroid use, and disease type), baseline variables significantly

© The Author(s), under exclusive license to Springer Nature Switzerland AG 2025
D. Colibaseanu et al., *Essential Articles in Colorectal Surgery*,
https://doi.org/10.1007/978-3-031-77745-5_3

associated ($P < .05$) with any infection or SSI separately, and TNFi exposure status. Exploratory models used TNFi exposure based on serum drug concentration.

Results: A total of 947 patients were enrolled from September 2014 through June 2017. Current TNFi exposure was reported by 382 patients. Any infection (18.1% vs. 20.2%, P = .469) and SSI (12.0% vs. 12.6%, P = .889) rates were similar in patients currently exposed to TNFis and those unexposed. In multivariable analysis, current TNFi exposure was not associated with any infection (odds ratio, 1.050; 95% confidence interval, 0.716–1.535) or SSI (odds ratio, 1.249; 95% confidence interval, 0.793–1.960). Detectable TNFi drug concentration was not associated with any infection or SSI.

Conclusions: Preoperative TNFi exposure was not associated with postoperative infectious complications in a large prospective multicenter cohort.

LS

This large prospective, multicenter study determined the absence of a relationship between the use of tumor necrosis factor inhibitors (TNFi) within 12 weeks of abdominal surgery for inflammatory bowel disease (IBD) and development of postoperative surgical site infections (SSIs). A total of 947 patients were enrolled in 17 participating sites over less than 3 years, which is remarkable. Serum drug levels were prospectively obtained for both infliximab and adalimumab. The study included a variety of surgical procedures, minimally invasive or open, involving any segment of the intestinal tract and requiring or not the creation of a stoma. All IBD diagnoses and disease phenotypes were included, ranging from ulcerative colitis to Crohn's disease to indeterminate colitis. SSI rates were significantly associated with preoperative use of corticosteroids, prior bowel resection, diabetes, hypertension, and smoking at the time of the intervention. Smoking and preoperative use of steroids were associated with the most significant odd ratios in the multivariate analysis. This study has provided clarity on the perioperative risks associated with TNFi and reassured surgeons about the safety of this class of medications. This is a practice-changing study. Previous single institutional reports had raised concerns associated with the risk of postoperative infections in patients receiving TNFi who underwent ileocolic resection, which could be offset by the creation of a diverting stoma [1]. In this area, it has been traditionally difficult to analyze the individual impact of biologic medications in patients in whom several other recognized risk factors for infections can coexist such as steroid use or malnutrition. Based on the PUCCINI results I feel that a systematic stoma diversion among TNFi users undergoing resection for Crohn's disease would be too Draconian. The many different operations included in the study truly reflect the real world but were also very heterogeneous. This renders it underpowered to draw definitive conclusions about the use of TNFi at the time of ileal pouch-anal anastomosis. For this particular indication, I still believe that patients on TNFi should undergo an initial total abdominal colectomy with end ileostomy, then discontinue the use of biologics, and return to the operative room after a few months for completion proctectomy and ileal pouch-anal anastomosis. There is retrospective data indicating that such staging of the surgical procedures is associated with a reduction of SSI rates when compared with patients who underwent upfront total proctocolectomy and ileal pouch-anal anastomosis while on infliximab [2]. The other consideration which is germane to this study is that the introduction of new biologic medications into the market largely outpaces the ability of any independent investigators to timely assess their specific risk of postoperative SSI. Even assuming a patient accrual as efficient as in the PUCCINI study, it would take years to obtain comparable data for each new biologic medication on the market. We therefore de facto assume that based on the PUCCINI results, all other biologics should be similarly safe without relying on an equally substantial body of evidence. While belonging to the same broad medication class, the mechanisms of action differ among biologic medications, and a specific agent could in theory be associated with increased postoperative SSI risk. There is some evidence, perhaps not as strong as this study, indicating that at least some of the other biologics are not associated with increased risk of postoperative SSIs. In any case, given their proven benefit in the medical management of IBD patients, we are inevitably faced with the dilemma of perioperative management of new medications, until they will have, if ever, their PUCCINI's equivalents.

References

1. Appau KA, Fazio VW, Shen B, Church JM, Lashner B, Remzi F, Brzezinski A, Strong SA, Hammel J, Kiran RP. Use of infliximab within 3 months of ileocolonic resection is associated with adverse postoperative outcomes in Crohn's patients. J Gastrointest Surg. 2008;12(10):1738–44.
2. Gu J, Remzi FH, Shen B, Vogel JD, Kiran RP. Operative strategy modifies risk of pouch-related outcomes in patients with ulcerative colitis on preoperative anti-tumor necrosis factor-α therapy. Dis Colon Rectum. 2013;56(11):1243–52.

Discussion

LS

This has changed my practice because I used to divert all patients who were on treatment with a biologic medication, and now, I no longer consider diversion only because somebody is on biologics. I ask patients to perhaps try and plan their operation relatively late after they receive their biologic medications so that we operate during a presumed nadir of the blood concentration of that specific medication, but that is all I do. And when this is impossible, I have still created undiverted anastomoses while presumably the blood concentration of the biologic medication was relatively high.

AM

I think when we look at this IBD population on biologics, the most significant impact on postoperative outcomes, in my opinion, does not come from being on anti-TNF. It is two other factors, which would be steroid use and malnutrition, and those probably have a far bigger impact on their outcome. I think the other thing that we need to consider practically is combination therapy or a combination of these risk factors. And so probably any one of these in isolation is far lesser of a factor than, for example, prednisone and malnutrition, which may be more severe, but I think you also have to consider the patient population treated with biologics and prednisone because these are probably markers of more severe disease, perhaps penetrating disease, which we know has an increased baseline risk of an anastomotic leak. But in general, I think the PUCCINI trial confirmed with far better data what we had seen historically in the Mayo Clinic literature which was that operating on biologics in the setting of Crohn's disease did not necessarily impart an increased complication risk, but in the setting of UC and J pouch, it did. Now, I think the other part, in response to your comment on J Pouch, Luca, is the fact that we are comparing completely different operations. In terms of commonality, I mean ileocolic resection at baseline, whether in a completely normal, healthy patient, or with relevant comorbidities is quite different than a low pelvic anastomosis, and that is where I think understanding the impact on biologics in J Pouch for UC will be far more difficult because of the risk profile of the operation at baseline. And so generally with such a high-stakes operation with not much of a fallback approach, if you were to encounter a significant complication like a leak, it is probably best to be more conservative and approach these in three stages for those patients on biologics.

MD

Considering the wide range of operations included in this study, as both of you mentioned, I still have concerns regarding the risk of biologics associated with J pouch surgery, particularly given the significant potential for permanent ileostomy in patients who experience a leak and pelvic sepsis. Therefore, while this study contributes to the broader discussion on the use of biologics in surgery, it may not directly address concerns specific to J pouch procedures. Additionally, it underscores the benefits of a three-staged approach, allowing patients to undergo full optimization prior to pouch creation, including considerations such as nutrition, smoking cessation, and discontinuation of all immunosuppressive medications. This approach likely plays a crucial role in reducing the risk of leak and pelvic sepsis. Furthermore, considering the evidence supporting a modified two-stage pouch, it suggests that pre-pouch optimization with cessation of all immunosuppressants may be the key factor in minimizing complications, rather than fecal diversion at the time of pouch creation.

DC

Great question, and great timing given what we knew at the time. A big reason why I think they did this study was that there were two French studies that looked at this question and had contradictory results. So, this was a bigger study, and I think that it helped clarify that question about the anti-TNF. What I found interesting about the study is that it did identify that having steroids on board is associated with a higher risk of postoperative infections, which was defined more broadly than just surgical site infections and adverse outcomes, but also diabetes, with odds ratio of 3.31, and the corresponding p value was 0.004, which is also concerning from my standpoint. Those are the two things that I took away from the paper, in addition to the fact that anti-TNF medications on their own are not independently associated with surgical site infection unlike having diabetes, for example. That should make us pause and see if we can actually control diabetes prior to surgery so that might be something to pay attention to. I think it was an interesting study, and it does change our practices or at least reinforces something that we already thought about doing—it is a well done, valuable study.

AM

I think one other comment is that I do not think we know in certain terms, but we're probably overall operating more frequently on Crohn's patients on biologics without stopping them. But I wonder if this has changed or increased rates of proximal diversion in these settings, because this is another thing that I think is very institutionally and culturally dependent, at least in terms of our training paradigms. Are there data on the role of diversion and intra-abdominal anastomosis, that is, diverting loop ileostomy vs. end ileostomy or just surgery without proximal diversion? Maybe these data exist, and I just have not seen them. What are the rates of proximal diversion or rates of non-anastomosis, just end ileostomy, among patients undergoing ileocolic resection for Crohn's post-PUCCINI trial? I do not know if those data exist.

LS

I do not know of any papers about it.

AM

Historically, the cultural training paradigm and thought at Mayo Clinic is that for intra-abdominal anastomosis, we tend not to divert. You either put the bowel segments together or you do not. I mean, I should say divert with a proximal loop ileostomy. You either put them together or you create an end ileostomy. The principle behind it is that the leak from an intra-abdominal anastomosis is not as contained or mitigated with a loop ileostomy when compared to a pelvic anastomosis.

LS

Yes, there is a school of thought along the same lines from Europe, and there are some publications which I did not include in the references. They advocate to put the colon and the ileum through the same opening, so the surgeons create at once an end ileostomy but also the setting for subsequent take down without a major laparotomy. They feel this approach gives the benefits of both the diverting loop ileostomy and end ileostomy based on what you were saying.

AM

That is what I do. Technically, even now. For example, after a right colon resection instead of putting the ileum and the colon together with a proximal loop ileostomy, I will try and bring them out through the same opening, or if I cannot because of body habitus or what not, I will tag the proximal colon right next to the stoma just beneath the fascia. So, I can get it through a peristomal incision, and it avoids a major laparotomy. And that makes sense; I think, I have done it.

LS

I agree that makes sense. I think I have done it twice in my career. However, I have done it only for patients who underwent reoperation for an abdominal anastomotic leak. I just feel more comfortable closing a diverting loop ileostomy than doing that. I understand the concern on the intra-abdominal anastomosis, but I have not often seen leaks from the defunctionalized ileocolic anastomosis, so this has remained as a personal habit of mine.

Is Early Surgery for Crohn's Disease Preferable to Continued Anti-TNFα Management?

4

Ponsioen CY, de Groof EJ, Eshuis EJ, Gardenbroek TJ, Bossuyt PMM, Hart A, Warusavitarne J, Buskens CJ, van Bodegraven AA, Brink MA, Consten ECJ, van Wagensveld BA, Rijk MCM, Crolla RMPH, Noomen CG, Houdijk APJ, Mallant RC, Boom M, Marsman WA, Stockmann HB, Mol B, de Groof AJ, Stokkers PC, D'Haens GR, Bemelman WA, LIR!C study group. Laparoscopic ileocaecal resection versus infliximab for terminal ileitis in Crohn's disease: a randomised controlled, open-label, multicentre trial. Lancet Gastroenterol Hepatol. 2017;2(11):785–92.

Abstract

Background: Treatment of patients with ileocecal Crohn's disease who have not responded to conventional therapy is commonly scaled up to biological agents, but surgery can also offer excellent short-term and long-term results. We compared laparoscopic ileocecal resection with infliximab to assess how they affect health-related quality of life.

Methods: In this randomized controlled, open-label trial, in 29 teaching hospitals and tertiary care centers in the Netherlands and the UK, adults with non-stricturing, ileocecal Crohn's disease, in whom conventional therapy has failed were randomly allocated (1:1) by an Internet randomization module with biased-coin minimization for participating centers and perianal fistula to receive laparoscopic ileocecal resection or infliximab. Eligible patients

© The Author(s), under exclusive license to Springer Nature Switzerland AG 2025
D. Colibaseanu et al., *Essential Articles in Colorectal Surgery*,
https://doi.org/10.1007/978-3-031-77745-5_4

23

were aged 18–80 years, had active Crohn's disease of the terminal ileum, and had not responded to at least 3 months of conventional therapy with glucocorticosteroids, thiopurines, or methotrexate. Patients with diseased terminal ileum longer than 40 cm or abdominal abscesses were excluded. The primary outcome was quality of life on the Inflammatory Bowel Disease Questionnaire (IBDQ) at 12 months. Secondary outcomes were general quality of life, measured by the Short Form-36 (SF-36) health survey and its physical and mental component subscales, days unable to participate in social life, days on sick leave, morbidity (additional procedures and hospital admissions), and body image and cosmesis. Analyses of the primary outcome were done in the intention-to-treat population, and safety analyses were done in the per-protocol population. This trial is registered at the Dutch Trial Registry (NTR1150).

Findings: Between May 2, 2008, and October 14, 2015, 73 patients were allocated to have resection and 70 to receive infliximab. Corrected for baseline differences, the mean IBDQ score at 12 months was 178.1 (95% CI 171.1–185.0) in the resection group versus 172.0 (164.3–179.6) in the infliximab group (mean difference 6.1 points, 95% CI –4.2 to 16.4; $p = 0.25$). At 12 months, the mean SF-36 total score was 112.1 (95% CI 108.0–116.2) in the resection group versus 106.5 (102.1–110.9) in the infliximab group (mean difference 5.6, 95% CI –0.4 to 11.6), the mean physical component score was 47.7 (45.7–49.7) versus 44.6 (42.5–46.8; mean difference 3.1, 4.2 to 6.0), and the mean mental component score was 49.5 (47.0–52.1) versus 46.1 (43.3–48.9; mean difference 3.5, –0.3 to 7.3). Mean numbers of days of sick leave were 3.4 days (SD 7.1) in the resection group versus 1.4 days (4.7) in the infliximab group ($p < 0.0001$), days not able to take part in social life were 1.8 days (6.3) versus 1.1 days (4.5; $p = 0.20$), days of scheduled hospital admission were 6.5 days (3.8) versus 6.8 days (3.2; $p = 0.84$), and the number of patients who had unscheduled hospital admissions were 13 (18%) of 73 versus 15 (21%) of 70 ($p = 0.68$). Body-image scale mean scores in the patients who had resection were 16.0 (95% CI 15.2–16.8) at baseline versus 17.8 (17.1–18.4) at 12 months, and cosmetic scale mean scores were 17.6 (16.6–18.6) versus 18.6 (17.6–19.6). Surgical intervention-related complications classified as IIIa or worse on the Clavien-Dindo scale occurred in four patients in the resection group. Treatment-related serious adverse events occurred in two patients in the infliximab group. During a median follow-up of 4 years (IQR 2–6), 26 (37%) of 70 patients in the infliximab group had resection, and 19 (26%) of 73 patients in the resection group received anti-TNF.

Interpretation: Laparoscopic resection in patients with limited (diseased terminal ileum <40 cm), non-stricturing, ileocecal Crohn's disease in whom conventional therapy has failed could be considered a reasonable alternative to infliximab therapy.

LS

Many surgeons treating inflammatory bowel disease are referred patients who have tried a multitude of medications for Crohn's disease with the idea of controlling their symptoms while avoiding surgery. They eventually capitulate and undergo surgery only to say after they recover that they wish they had done surgery earlier. The investigators of the LIR!C trial could actually design a study where the option of early surgery for terminal ileal disease could be examined in a rigorous fashion. Patients with terminal ileal Crohn's disease were randomized to have laparoscopic surgery vs. escalation of medical management to infliximab following failure of at least 3 months of what was described as conventional therapy with steroids, thiopurines, or methotrexate. A diseased segment longer than 40 cm, previous ileocolic resection, penetrating phenotype, or stricturing phenotype indicated by prestenotic bowel dilatation constituted a contraindication to study enrollment. The primary aim was comparing quality-of-life measures through widely accepted questionnaires, and all relevant quality-of-life scores were comparable between the groups. Adverse events related to the respective treatments were also comparable. Long-term results based on 94% of the original study population having a median follow-up of 63.5 months provided further support for early laparoscopic ileocolic resection as a suitable treatment option in this patient population. None of the patients originally randomized to surgery required a second resection, while 48% of the patients originally randomized to infliximab ended up requiring a resection. Duration of treatment effect was comparable between the groups [1]. One aspect of the study which I would find difficult to replicate in my practice is that the investigators of the LIR!C study specifically selected inflammatory disease phenotype and excluded stricturing phenotype. Besides patients with prestenotic ileal dilatation, they also excluded patients with an absence of inflammation on screening magnetic resonance enterography. Our radiology department has considerable experience with magnetic resonance imaging, but I think it is often difficult to separately identify the components of inflammation versus fibrosis in terminal ileal disease. The majority of patients who we are asked to evaluate generally have some form of a stricture, not necessarily with an identifiable proximal dilatation but some degree of stricture nonetheless based on radiology and/or endoscopy. They generally come to see me when they have already been started on biologics, and sometimes, their disease has symptomatically responded to biologics despite previously documented strictures. I feel the separation of inflammatory tissue from fibrotic tissue to identify who needs surgery and who could respond to medical management remains a sort of Holy Grail. In addition, there are patients who could swear that with some adjustments, their quality of life is acceptable, while they have terrible radiological or endoscopic findings. It is uncommon to discuss surgery with a patient that has clearly and only inflammatory disease phenotype. This is in a way a limitation of the present study but at the same time reveals exceptional skills in designing a complex study and indicates an open culture where all treatment options are assessed fairly in their advantages and disadvantages. It is obvious that most patients do not like the idea of surgery, and it is not intuitive that a patient would prefer to have early surgery rather than medical management. In addition, if 48% of patients on infliximab required surgery after 5 years, this means that 52% could do without it. The benefits of early surgery for terminal ileal Crohn's disease on long-term outcomes remain controversial [2, 3]. However, the results of the LIR!C trial are important because they foster an evolutionary change in our culture which influences surgeons and gastroenterologists alike. It is still inconceivable to recommend surgery to each and every patient with terminal ileitis who fails first-line medical management. However, it is increasingly accepted that a discussion on early surgery makes sense and could become the preferred option in the individual patient.

References

1. Stevens TW, Haasnoot ML, D'Haens GR, Buskens CJ, de Groof EJ, Eshuis EJ, Gardenbroek TJ, Mol B, Stokkers PCF, Bemelman WA, Ponsioen CY, LIR!C study group. Laparoscopic ileocaecal resection versus infliximab for terminal ileitis in Crohn's disease: retrospective long-term follow-up of the LIR!C trial. Lancet Gastroenterol Hepatol. 2020;5(10):900–7.
2. Beelen EMJ, Arkenbosch JHC, Erler NS, Sleutjes JAM, Hoentjen F, Bodelier AGL, Dijkstra G, Romberg-Camps M, de Boer NK, Stassen LPS, van der Meulen AE, West R, van Ruler O, van der Woude CJ, de Vries AC. Impact of timing of primary ileocecal resection on prognosis in patients with Crohn's disease. BJS Open. 2023;7(5):zrad097.
3. Agrawal M, Ebert AC, Poulsen G, Ungaro RC, Faye AS, Jess T, Colombel JF, Allin KH. Early ileocecal resection for Crohn's disease is associated with improved long-term outcomes compared with anti-tumor necrosis factor therapy: a population-based cohort study. Gastroenterology. 2023;165(4):976–85.e3.

Discussion

LS

I admire to the point of envy what this group of investigators accomplished because it is one thing that I thought about for many years, but I could never find a way of doing a study to prove it. I think this study has influenced the opinion of gastroenterologists about surgery. As a surgeon, I have noticed that at least some gastroenterologists are more comfortable in using surgery as a treatment option in the appropriate patient instead of persisting in the use of medications. This is particularly the case for younger patients with good nutritional status and no history of steroid use who are at low risk of perioperative complications. This subset of patients can undergo an ileocolic resection and primary anastomosis, really restart the clock on the natural history of their disease, and potentially respond better to medical management with a decreased burden of disease. Many of the patients similar to those included in this study could respond to medical treatment so that surgery can be delayed, but it is otherwise inevitable. It becomes a sort of kicking the can. Many gastroenterologists are now much more liberal in recommending surgery to their patients and that facilitates my job as a surgeon. I do not like to be in the position of having to convince anybody on the appropriateness of surgery.

AM

I think that not just with ileocolic disease, but throughout the surgical care of IBD, we have never seen surgery as a failure and rather as a critical element in the continuum of the patient's care. I think this study has perhaps allowed some gastroenterologists to accept the fact that surgery does not constitute failure of care. I feel strongly, and even prior to this study, but based on poorer quality literature, that early surgery in a subset of IBD patients, Crohn's in particular, is far more beneficial than, as you said, kicking the can down the road. This is a much better situation than having someone sustained on multiple biologics and multiple exposures to these medications for a long period of time where now you are faced with operating on them. Or maybe not just on multiple immunosuppressants but also now malnourished, with the addition of prednisone, because they try and control the disease as much as possible prior to opening the door for the surgeon to see and counsel the patient. Fundamentally, gastroenterologists are the gatekeepers of this patient population, and I think this will always be a struggle in terms of getting the surgical message out there.

MD

This study has certainly led to more frequent opportunities for intervention. However, I must point out that the patient population in this study does not reflect those we typically encounter in our surgical clinics. When we discuss deferring intervention or "kicking the can down the road," we are often dealing with patients who have exhausted multiple biologics, experienced admissions for obstructions, or present with more severe disease manifestations such as stricturing or penetrating disease, a patient population that was not studied in this paper. The study demonstrates considerable success with medical management alone, in a highly selective group of patients with mild disease. In this patient population, half of the patients did not require surgery and showed signs of improvement while on Remicade, with many achieving endoscopic response as well. While this suggests that surgery could be considered as an initial treatment option, it does not necessarily imply that it is a superior one.

AM

That is almost by the necessity of trial design, right? You really need to have a patient population that has early disease to compare to. Otherwise, if you are selecting those that have more advanced disease, to me, at least it would not be as clear of a comparison of surgery to initiating medical treatment. If you have a patient who already has fibrotic disease, we know, with very good data, that no medication is going to help that patient. So, almost by necessity, you had to select the patients with early disease—a disease that just looks inflammatory to ask: is surgery as complicated when compared to medical management?

MD

I agree, but this study does not indicate that surgery is inherently superior to medical management for this specific patient demographic. Instead, it highlights a shift in perspective particularly for our gastroenterology colleagues, where early surgical intervention is becoming more acceptable, particularly for patients who may have reservations about long-term medication use. I think it is important to note that this study does not imply that medical management is no longer a first-line option for these patients. I think both surgical and medical approaches have their place, and the decision should be tailored to individual patient needs and preferences.

LS

A total of 48% of patients randomized to infliximab ended up requiring surgery. And so, I think this also speaks to the "kicking the can" concept. And of course, you could argue that 52% did not require surgery. I agree with you, but among patients who ended up having surgery, I wonder if their quality of life was miserable during those intervening years. How well did they really do in those years where they did not have surgery or did they really do well with medical management and could avoid surgery for a few years, which could make sense? I think you are right, the study does not condemn medical management, but it also stimulates the idea of selecting those patients who should be recommended to have surgery earlier.

AM

I just need to mention that the medication group was different than the surgical group. If I recall, those in the infliximab group had a higher incidence of perianal disease, so are they getting escalated on medications for different reasons that do not concern the primary site? So, the question is whether they were on medical therapy more frequently than the surgical group, perhaps because they have disease at a different site.

MD

Is this study changing your practice significantly? If you have a patient that comes in with mild inflammatory disease would you strongly recommend surgery over medical management?

LS

Well, no. I mean, not strongly. This is currently more of a theoretical scenario rather than a practical scenario given the realistic disease presentations we are faced with, as we mentioned before. Given the circumstances, I feel I would not recommend surgery strongly, but I would openly talk about the natural history of disease and quality of life, especially in young patients. It is reassuring to know that there are data which can help me in that discussion. The other practical issue in this conversation is that oftentimes patients come in with a preset opinion about surgery, which can be favorable or unfavorable. I oftentimes feel that we are a sort of a product located on a shelf and we are picked up based on the patient's own preference. Some of these preconceived ideas can be prejudicial against surgery. It is not common that the patient just comes in asking us for advice given our expertise in the treatment of their disease. In those circumstances, there is no point in presenting, explaining, or defending the literature. If requested, I could certainly quote the LIR!C trial as evidence supporting surgery, but I have to confess that I tend to go with the flow. I present my opinion understanding that mine is just one opinion among many.

AM

Yes, again, I think it is symbolic of how gastroenterologists remain the gatekeepers of the disease. We are partners, I think, perhaps unfortunately, lesser partners sometimes in the treatment decisions. To answer your question, for me, maybe I push it a little bit harder, but I think this paper has given us at least a platform to present more robust data that say that patients can do equally as well as those on medications. Also, to some patients, the side effects of medications are concerning enough to proceed with surgery. Or maybe it is for the younger patients who are looking at medical treatment over a much longer period of time. Maybe surgery can give them a number of years prior to even initiating a biologic, or maybe it is just immunomodulator therapy to save exposure to the biologic for a later date.

LS

Dorin, did the LIR!C study change your practice?

DC

Not much. I think probably because I already had a similar bias. Before we look at the study itself, there is an important question of how the disease phenotype is determined to be stricturing vs. non-stricturing. They try to describe it, but essentially, what they say is that patients are excluded if they had previously ileocecal resection or obstructive Crohn's at the terminal ileum that would probably require surgery. So, when you take that into account, the fact that this was a multi-institutional study, both in the Netherlands and in the UK, and you take into account a number of radiologists and endoscopists that are assessing whether this is inflammatory or not, then we have to take that with a grain of salt. We add to that the fact that even though roughly about 70 patients were assigned in each group at the beginning, we actually end up with more patients having surgery, 13 individuals who failed medical management, and so even though the groups didn't change a lot with the intention-to-treat design, what actually ended up happening is still that 13 patients failed infliximab treatment and required surgery. So, I think that all this points out to the fact that earlier surgery is not detrimental, and it is probably going to help the patient. That was the impression I had before but that was based on the fact that at least in my mind, inflammation and stricturing disease are not at all separate processes, but separate points along a continuum of disease progression; we just frequently do not know where we are on that continuum despite MRI, endoscopic assessment, with the exception of obvious stricturing disease. We do not know if it is just inflammation or if there is some stricturing as well. That is a long-winded way of saying that it did not change my practice and that probably I favor surgery earlier.

Stapled vs. Handsewn Ileal Pouch-Anal Anastomosis for Ulcerative Colitis

5

Ziv Y, Fazio VW, Church JM, Lavery IC, King TM, Ambrosetti P. Stapled ileal pouch anal anastomoses are safer than handsewn anastomoses in patients with ulcerative colitis. Am J Surg. 1996;171(3):320–3.

Abstract

Background: One of the theoretic advantages of using a stapled versus handsewn ileal pouch-anal anastomosis (IPAA) in restorative proctocolectomy is a reduction in septic complications. We performed this study to compare the incidence of early septic complications in patients undergoing restorative proctocolectomy with stapled or handsewn IPAA.

Patients and Methods: A chart review of 692 patients undergoing restorative proctocolectomy for treatment of ulcerative colitis was performed. The incidence of early septic complications in patients having stapled IPAA was compared to that in patients having handsewn IPAA. Follow-up studies included an annual questionnaire and physical examination.

Results: Of the 692 patients, 238 had handsewn IPAA and 454 had stapled IPAA; these two groups were similar in sex, duration of disease, age at surgery, and type of surgical procedure performed. In the handsewn IPAA group, 25 patients (10.5%) had 32 septic complications, and 24 required 89 reparations. In 7 patients, the pouch was excised. In the stapled IPAA group, 21 patients

© The Author(s), under exclusive license to Springer Nature Switzerland AG 2025
D. Colibaseanu et al., *Essential Articles in Colorectal Surgery*,
https://doi.org/10.1007/978-3-031-77745-5_5

(4.6%) had 23 septic complications, and 14 required 40 reparations. One patient needed pouch excision. There were more patients ($P = 0.0001$) with early septic complications, and more ($P < 0.0001$) pouch excisions because of these complications, in patients with handsewn IPAA than in patients with stapled IPAA. The sepsis-related reoperation rates did not differ significantly.

Conclusions: The stapled technique for IPAA has fewer septic complications and results in fewer sepsis-related pouch excisions, in our hands, than the handsewn technique, for treating patients with ulcerative colitis.

LS

This is a study which did not have the strongest methodological design but was convincing in that it came from a unit with extensive experience in ileal pouch-anal anastomosis. A stapled technique is intuitively easier than a handsewn technique, and the results of this study were not surprising. The other recognized advantage of stapled ileal pouch-anal anastomosis not specifically addressed by this study is in its functional outcomes. An earlier prospective randomized study with a smaller number of patients failed to detect a significant difference between mucosectomy and handsewn anastomosis versus stapled anastomosis [1]. However, subsequent experiences have corroborated the functional advantages associated with the stapled approach which has established itself as the preferred ileal pouch-anal anastomotic technique. In a metanalysis on 8872 patients (4871 patients in the stapled group and 4038 in the handsewn group) included in 31 studies, the stapled group had a lower rate of anastomotic stricture, small bowel obstruction, and ileal pouch failure. Operative times, anastomotic leak, pelvic sepsis, pouchitis rates, and hospital stays were similar. With respect to functional outcomes, the stapled group was associated with reduced rates of seepage, both during day and night times, pad use, and night incontinence [2]. One of the putative reasons to perform a mucosectomy would be the complete removal of the inflamed tissue to prevent the subsequent onset of cancer. However, older studies have indicated that even after mucosectomy, small islets of rectal mucosa and anal glands can remain [3], and therefore, it is not surprising that a considerable proportion of patients who develop cancer of the ileal pouch-anal anastomosis had indeed undergone mucosectomy which therefore should not be considered as protective for the onset of cancer. On the other hand, a retained anorectal cuff can allow more effective detection of abnormalities including dysplasia during long-term surveillance after ileal pouch-anal anastomosis. The above-mentioned metanalysis indicated no difference between the two groups in terms of dysplasia and neoplasia. Stapled anastomosis can undergo surveillance safely, and dysplasia in the anal transitional zone does not automatically require mucosectomy or pouch excision [4]. An elective indication for mucosectomy and hand-sewn ileal pouch-anal anastomosis is cancer of the rectum in the background of ulcerative colitis, especially if located in the distal third of the viscus. Colorectal dysplasia without cancer or cancer in the more proximal rectum is a more controversial indication. Otherwise, most surgeons treating ulcerative colitis in this day and age perform stapled ileal pouch-anal anastomosis.

References

1. Reilly WT, Pemberton JH, Wolff BG, Nivatvongs S, Devine RM, Litchy WJ, McIntyre PB. Randomized prospective trial comparing ileal pouch-anal anastomosis performed by excising the anal mucosa to ileal pouch-anal anastomosis performed by preserving the anal mucosa. Ann Surg. 1997;225(6):666–76; discussion 676–7.
2. Chaouch MA, Hussain MI, Gouader A, Krimi B, Mazzotta A, Costa ACD, Petrucciani N, Bouassida M, Khan J, Noomen F, Oweira H. Stapled anastomosis versus hand-sewn anastomosis with mucosectomy for ileal pouch-anal anastomosis: a systematic review and meta-analysis of postoperative outcomes, functional outcomes, and oncological safety. Cancer Control. 2024;31:10732748241236338.

3. O'Connell PR, Pemberton JH, Weiland LH, Beart RW Jr, Dozois RR, Wolff BG, Telander RL. Does rectal mucosa regenerate after ileoanal anastomosis? Dis Colon Rectum. 1987;30(1):1–5.
4. Silva-Velazco J, Stocchi L, Wu XR, Shen B, Remzi FH. Twenty-year-old stapled pouches for ulcerative colitis without evidence of rectal cancer: implications for surveillance strategy? Dis Colon Rectum. 2014;57(11):1275–81.

Discussion

DC

Excellent study; it is almost 30 years old, with almost 700 patients. Excellent question, especially at the time, and I think they answered reasonably well, especially being able to now in retrospect see that most pouches today by far are stapled. Fundamentally, a handsewn anastomosis is going to be lower, will take longer, and will be more difficult. There are certainly circumstances where it is warranted, but for me, stapled is the way to go.

LS

I think what was impressive to me in this study is that it was published during a period where there was a debate on the best anastomotic technique, and this study is definitely in favor of stapled anastomosis, while a prospective randomized trial that was done at the same time was inconclusive. Besides the individual characteristics of each study, this is a situation where in retrospect, it feels as if a study with a worse methodological design ultimately advocates for something that becomes the preferred standard of care, which is the stapled ileal pouch-anal anastomosis and particularly with the recognized advantages in anal function compared to the handsewn anastomosis. I think that there are very few advocates of systematic handsewn anastomosis for this indication in general whereas, clearly, the original technique description included handsewn technique, and there used to be a time when stapled anastomosis was introduced when there was a lot of debate. The other hypothesis which, I think, is widely considered as debunked today is the idea that with a mucosectomy, we can completely remove the diseased mucosa. Instead, we can see that in those rare but possible cancers which can occur at the ileal pouch-anal anastomosis, mucosectomy is not protective, and there are cells that could lead to cancer which are left in place even after handsewn anastomosis which was also demonstrated by specific studies examining pathologic specimen of removed ileal pouches.

DC

Luca, do you think that this might be one of those "lost arts"? Could it be that the technique is lost, so to speak? Just like we do not do anymore "S" pouches. I have learned how to do it, but I do not do them anymore.

LS

We do so much less handsewn anastomoses in general, so I think that you might be right, but I think the reason stapled anastomosis is preferable is that functional results are better, and there's pretty strong evidence indicating that it is basically safe for the risk of cancer in the retained cuff. It might seem counterintuitive that patients do better while retaining disease in place in the anal transitional zone, so I understand the argument in the abstract, but now, there are thousands of patients that have had stapled anastomosis providing compelling data on postoperative outcomes, risk of dysplasia, cancer, and long-term functional results. I think there is no point in doing a study indicating, for example, how many of the handsewn anastomoses develop anastomotic structure. My impression is that I have seen in the office over the years a lot of patients with 30-year-old pouches who have symptomatic strictures, and I do not feel that I see as many patients who have strictures after stapled anastomosis. So, to me, the verdict is clearly in favor of stapled technique. Of course, there are situations where handsewn can be preferable, I am thinking of dysplasia in the anal transitional zone or perhaps cancer in the low rectum. However, these are not common situations.

MD

I agree with all the comments. I think this was a very impressive paper by sheer numbers alone. And that, yes, I think that there's really no further controversy with regard to handsewn vs. stapled. I think that the one nice thing or the one thing that handsewn offers is that you do not have the concern about retained rectum. I think with regard to stapled pouches, some rectal cuffs are left too long, which can ultimately lead to problems with the pouch or ongoing proctitis, even after the pouch operation due to retained rectal cuff. In some cases, the surgeon may feel certain that they are low enough, and they think they are about 2 cm, but in fact, they are anywhere between 4 and 6 cm from the anal verge. So that would be, I would say, the only advantage at this point, short of the specific scenarios that Luca, you were talking about.

Intentional Ileal Pouch-Anal Anastomosis for Crohn's Disease

6

Melton GB, Fazio VW, Kiran RP, He J, Lavery IC, Shen B, Achkar JP, Church JM, Remzi FH. Long-term outcomes with ileal pouch-anal anastomosis and Crohn's disease: pouch retention and implications of delayed diagnosis. Ann Surg. 2008;248(4):608–16.

Abstract

Objective: To assess long-term outcomes after ileal pouch-anal anastomosis (IPAA) in Crohn's disease (CD).

Summary of Background Data: While considered the procedure of choice for ulcerative colitis, performance of ileal pouch-anal anastomosis (IPAA) is controversial in CD.

Methods: CD patients were identified from a prospectively maintained IPAA database. Time-to-diagnosis and pouch retention rates were analyzed using Kaplan–Meier curves. Demographic, clinical, and pathologic factors associated with pouch retention were evaluated with log-rank test and Cox proportional hazards model.

Results: Two hundred and four CD patients (108 female, median age 33 years, and median follow-up 7.4 years) with primary IPAA were included. CD diagnosis was before IPAA (intentional) in 20 (10%), from postoperative histopathology (incidental) in 97 (47%) or made in a delayed fashion at median 36 months after IPAA in 87 (43%). Overall 10-year pouch retention was 71%. On multivariate analysis, pouch loss was associated with delayed diagnosis (P 0.03, hazard ratio HR 2.6 (95% confidence interval CI 1.1–6.5)), pouch-vaginal fistula (P 0.01, HR 2.8 (95% CI 1.3–6.4)), and pelvic sepsis (P 0.0001, HR 9.7 (95% CI 3.4–27.3)). Patients with retained IPAA at follow-up had near-perfect/perfect continence (72%), rare/no urgency (68%) with median daily bowel movements 7 (range 2–20). Median overall quality of life, quality of health, level of energy, and happiness with surgery were 9, 9, 8, and 10 of 10, respectively.

Conclusions: For CD patients with IPAA, when the diagnosis is established preoperatively or immediately following surgery, pouch loss rates are low and functional results are favorable. Outcomes in patients with delayed diagnosis are worse but half retain their pouch at 10 years with good functional outcomes.

LS

This is a fundamental paper in the assessment of the relationship between Crohn's disease (CD) and ileal pouch-anal anastomosis (IPAA). It provides some fundamental definitions which have helped my assessment of the disease under these circumstances. The authors analyzed a total of 204 patients with CD during a median follow-up of 7.4 years. This included 20 patients who had "intentional IPAA" with CD; that is, the IPAA was constructed on patients having a known preoperative diagnosis of CD. In 97 patients, the diagnosis of CD was made on the surgical specimen at the time of postoperative pathology evaluation, which was defined as "incidental IPAA" and CD. In the remaining 87 patients, the diagnosis of CD was made during follow-up, hence the term "delayed IPAA" and CD. The overall pouch retention rate was 71%, and it was significantly different when comparing the 85% rate associated with intentional IPAA and the 87% associated with incidental IPAA against the 53% rate in case of delayed diagnosis. Factors independently associated with pouch loss were delayed diagnosis, pouch-vaginal fistula, and pelvic sepsis, which is not surprising. For example, if a patient who had an IPAA with a diagnosis of ulcerative colitis develops pouch inflammation associated with multiple perianal fistulas several years after his or her index surgery, one would imagine that given this clinical scenario, this patient faces an increased risk of pouch loss. On the other hand, a high pouch retention rate associated with incidental IPAA for CD is also expected and consistent with previous reports. However, the results of intentional IPAA are more provocative in that they challenge the traditional assumption of CD as a contraindication to IPAA. The number of patients with intentional IPAA is small but reflects other experiences indicating that intentional IPAA is feasible in this subset of patients and is associated with acceptable pouch retention rates. A systematic review including 258 patients with CD diagnosed either before IPAA or based on surgical pathology at the time of proctocolectomy indicated a pouch failure rate of 15% after a mean follow-up of 69 months [1]. It is notable that patients in this series could be candidates for intentional IPAA for CD only if they had no CD in the small bowel or perianal CD. More recently, the largest experience to date of IPAA used intentionally for well-defined CD reported by Aviran and coll, also included patients with perianal Crohn's disease and small bowel disease. After a median follow-up of 93 months, 22 patients (48%) developed recurrent CD, but only four patients (9%) experienced pouch failure [2]. Intentional IPAA for CD is a topic which generates a lot of enthusiasm, and I would venture saying that I personally had more discussions about it than patients with it. Having said that, I feel that this is a small group of patients who tend to do relatively well after IPAA. It is often mentioned that this option should be offered to motivated patients. I feel that at least when applying the original selection criteria excluding perianal disease and small bowel disease, those who should be motivated in offering intentional IPAA for CD are the surgeons rather than the patients. On the other hand, considering patients with perianal disease and/or small bowel disease for intentional IPAA remains an aggressive approach, notwithstanding the excellent results presented by the Cedar Sinai group. This should be considered the cutting-edge application of intentional IPAA, recognizing that modern medical management has rendered increasingly feasible the management of recurrent Crohn's disease of the J pouch in its various manifestations. These are the cases where patient motivation and their acceptance of the significant risks associated with this approach are still essential.

References

1. Lightner AL, Jia X, Zaghiyan K, Fleshner PR. IPAA in known preoperative Crohn's disease: a systematic review. Dis Colon Rectum. 2021;64(3):355–64.
2. Aviran E, Assaf D, Zaghiyan K, Fleshner P. Long-term outcomes and factors predicting outcome of IPAA when used intentionally for well-defined Crohn's disease. Dis Colon Rectum. 2023;66(5):700–6.

Discussion

LS

The data from Cedar Sinai in Los Angeles is provocative in that they push the envelope much further than this particular paper because they have created intentional ileal pouches in patients who have anal fistulas and/or a history of small bowel disease and their patients have been able to retain most of their pouches. These would still be contraindications based on the criteria presented in this paper. The indications reported in this paper are now straightforward to me, but I am still hesitant to be as aggressive as the Cedar Sinai group.

MD

I agree. This paper provides valuable insights, especially considering its substantial sample size of over 200 patients, for a disease process that most institutions rarely see. It offers some reassurance when considering pouch surgery for this particular patient population, demonstrating that individuals with Crohn's disease can still fare well with a pouch despite their condition. One aspect I found intriguing was their differentiation between patients with a pre-existing diagnosis of Crohn's disease before pouch surgery versus those initially diagnosed with UC or indeterminate colitis who later developed Crohn's. The finding that those who developed Crohn's later on had worse outcomes is noteworthy. Despite the limitations of its retrospective and heterogeneous design, this paper provides compelling data supporting the consideration of a pouch in patients with Crohn's disease, particularly those without perianal or small bowel involvement.

LS

I think it relates to this idea of Crohn's disease of the ileal J pouch. A patient may have been diagnosed with ulcerative colitis based on both a colectomy and proctectomy specimens. Then, it is possible that several years after they had a J pouch, they start developing fistulas from the ileal pouch. They could be anal fistulas distal to the anastomosis that can be treated conservatively and/or pouch fistulas which are more likely to put the ileal pouch at risk. This phenomenon does occur, and I do discuss it as a risk when obtaining consent for ileal pouch-anal anastomosis. These patients unfortunately tend to declare themselves after the pouch is already done in which case the outcome will likely be worse.

DC

I think this paper at least encouraged me to consider patients with Crohns's who really insist on having a pouch. If they have never had anal disease, or fistulas, and they clearly understand what the risks are, I think I would engage in a discussion with them.

Revisionary Surgery for Failed Ileal Pouch-Anal Anastomosis

Remzi FH, Aytac E, Ashburn J, et al. Transabdominal redo ileal pouch surgery for failed restorative proctocolectomy: lessons learned over 500 patients. Ann Surg. 2015;262(4):675–82.

Abstract

Objectives: The purpose of this study was to report our large, single-center experience of transabdominal ileal pouch-anal anastomoses (IPAA) redo surgery for a failed initial IPAA.

Background: IPAA fail from 3% to 15% of the times, mainly due to technical or inflammatory conditions. There is limited information about the surgical, functional, and quality-of-life (QOL) outcomes of redo surgery for failed IPAA, especially in large series of patients.

Methods: Patients undergoing transabdominal redo surgery for failed IPAA between 1983 and 2014 were evaluated. Primary endpoints were morbidity of the surgery, the proportion of patients with a functioning pouch, frequency of defecation and incidence of incontinence, and the patients' perception of QOL.

Results: There were 502 (43% males) patients with a median age of 38 years and median body mass index of 24 kg/m^2 at the time of revision surgery. A new pouch was created in 41% of patients, whereas 59% had their original pouch revised and retained. Postoperative mortality was 0% and morbidity was 53%. The short-term anastomotic leak rate was 8%. At a median

© The Author(s), under exclusive license to Springer Nature Switzerland AG 2025

D. Colibaseanu et al., *Essential Articles in Colorectal Surgery*, https://doi.org/10.1007/978-3-031-77745-5_7

follow-up of 7 years after redo surgery, 101 (n = 20%) patients had redo IPAA failure. Pelvic sepsis developing after redo ileal pouch surgery was the primary indicator of pouch failure (hazard ratio, 3.691; 95% confidence interval, 2.411–5.699; $P < 0.0001$). Overall functional outcomes and QOL scores were acceptable.

Conclusions: Patients with a failed ileoanal pouch may be offered redo pouch surgery with a high likelihood of success in terms of function and QOL.

LS

This is a large retrospective study from a group with extensive experience in managing complications of ileal pouch-anal anastomosis (IPAA). Its results indicate that revisionary pouch surgery can be successful in selected patients. However, the importance of selecting the right patient for these demanding operations cannot be overemphasized. This is the kind of operation which should not be prescribed to patients but rather discussed and chosen based on both appropriate indications but also individual patient preferences. It is possible that a patient who has already suffered for a long time following complications of his or her primary ileal pouch-anal anastomosis can also experience failure of revisionary pouch surgery and be condemned to ultimately accept an end ileostomy as his or her only option. Patient motivation in this clinical situation is therefore paramount. The other aspect that is very important is that many of these patients come to the discussion in severe distress caused by their dysfunctional ileal pouch, and an initial diverting ileostomy can control their symptoms and optimize them for their pelvic revisionary operation. In doing this, it is important to consider the consequences of the specific bowel loop that is selected to become a diverting loop ileostomy. Schwartzberg et al. have presented the concept of "thoughtful ileostomy," where the two limbs selected to become the diverting loop ileostomy under these circumstances could easily become the two limbs of a redo J pouch and reach the anus without tension should that become necessary [1]. One useful aspect in patient counseling which emerges from this paper and was confirmed by a subsequent publication from Toronto is that revisionary pouch surgery due to mechanical factors is associated with an increased probability of success when compared to redo pouch for pelvic sepsis or pouch-vaginal fistula [2]. A particular situation is that of a patient in whom an ileal pouch-anal anastomosis performed using minimally invasive technique [3] by an inexperienced surgeon has resulted in a long anorectal cuff and poor functional outcomes. On one hand, this is a preventable complication had the index operation been conducted in a technically appropriate fashion. On the other hand, this is a clinical situation where revisionary pouch surgery may be associated with limited pelvic adhesions so that a stapled ileal pouch-anal anastomosis at the level of the anorectal ring is possible using the original J pouch once the excess anorectal cuff has been trimmed off. This is a situation where revisionary pouch surgery can substantially help the patient. In the discussion of this paper at the time of its presentation, which is reported with the article, the senior author also emphasized the poor outcomes associated with redo pouch performed for pouchitis which should therefore be viewed as a contraindication. Despite its high success rate, revisionary pouch surgery remains associated with significant morbidity, and functional results vary. A multidisciplinary approach especially with active participation by gastroenterology and radiology is therefore critical. If this is not available, the patient should be probably referred to a center where multidisciplinary expertise is available.

References

1. Schwartzberg DM, Esen E, Remzi FH. Thoughtful ileostomy creation in patients undergoing redo IPAA. Dis Colon Rectum. 2020;63(1):117–20.
2. Pooni A, Brar MS, Kennedy E, Cohen Z, MacRae H, de Buck van Overstraeten A. Transabdominal IPAA revision: does indication dictate outcome? Dis Colon Rectum. 2023;66(4):559–66.

3. Aydinli HH, Esen E, Aytac E, Kirat HT, Schwartzberg DM, Chang S, Remzi FH. Transabdominal pouch salvage for failed minimally invasive versus open IPAA: a case-matched study. Dis Colon Rectum. 2020;63(8):1102–7.

Discussion

DC

This is pretty outstanding work with regards to 7 years of follow-up after redo pouch surgery. If you were to ask somebody, not having read the paper, what the failure rate of a redo pouch is, probably, people would think that the rate is higher than the 20% failure rate published in this paper. It is not great, obviously, but in the context that this is in a 20% failure rate is, I would say, a lot better than I would have thought prior to reading this paper. And this is in 2015, and I am sure that they are probably ready for an update anytime soon. Turning to you Luca, being one of the authors, my questions would be about the subsequent short gut. That is something that I always worry about. And then I also worry about reach in redo pouches. How much tougher it is if patients are big, etc.?

LS

I was one of the coauthors, but this is not my paper and largely results from many years of practice from a center with experience and a number of very skilled surgeons who preceded me or/and were more senior than me at the time. Short-gut syndrome is not really a common problem even in case of redo pouch failure; of course, high ileostomy output can be a vexing issue, but among those who are selected to undergo redo pouch, there should be a low risk of becoming truly TPN-dependent. I think as far as the BMI and this would be the same for comorbidities and general patient condition, the surgeon needs to be selective which I think is critical for success. Patients selected for redo pouch are frequently younger, and their BMI tends to be a little lower than patients for example who undergo surgery for primary rectal cancer. So, I think that it can be an issue, but less so than I think in other situations.

DC

When you do the pouch, and I am referring to kind of your personal experience, do you find that we have less of lengthening procedure options? There are not a lot of vessels we can additionally take when we redo. Or is there?

LS

If the ileocolic artery was not divided, this should be the first consideration; otherwise, there is not a prescriptive mesenteric vessel branch division approach of which I am aware. If mesenteric mobilization does not help reduce tension, then it might be possible to reconstruct an ileal pouch with the mesentery positioned anteriorly or create an S pouch or accept a smaller ileal pouch. Mesenteric windows can help. Having said that, an excision of the pouch and IPAA reconstruction with a new pouch can be very difficult because of tension, and the possible inability to reestablish intestinal continuity should be discussed with the patient preoperatively. However, there is also a subset of patients, who are amenable to revision of the existing pouch, and they may have a dilated, dysfunctional ileal pouch so that tension might not be really an issue. So, still very difficult case but not as problematic perhaps.

DC

Yes, it really sounds to me that the population of patients that come with pouch problems that need revision consists of a very heterogeneous set of problems. That is where that expertise comes in, because you are not getting many of the exact same types of issues, which require a lot of innovation, which should best be supported by a solid background of experience. I would say in cases of redo pouches I would probably ask Luca for help and not try to tackle them on my own.

LS

I also feel we should consider planning a combined case with our surgical partners for these difficult situations unless you are one of the few with vast experience in this.

We could lament the lack of skills of some surgeons who do primary ileal pouches without the necessary training and experience, but at the same time, I think it is very difficult in the United States due to the very fragmented healthcare. You have some community surgeons who serve their community, and you have patients who simply cannot afford to travel, so we cannot just blame the surgeon. There are other factors at play.

MD

I think to a certain extent it is inevitable in the current healthcare system.

Optimization of Rectal Cancer Surgery: The Concept of Total Mesorectal Excision

8

Heald RJ, Husband EM, Ryall RD. The mesorectum in rectal cancer surgery—the clue to pelvic recurrence? Br J Surg. 1982;69(10):613–6.

Abstract

Five cases are described where minute foci of adenocarcinoma have been demonstrated in the mesorectum several centimeters distal to the apparent lower edge of a rectal cancer. In two of these, there was no other evidence of lymphatic spread of the tumor. In orthodox anterior resection, much of this tissue remains in the pelvis, and it is suggested that these foci might lead to suture line or pelvic recurrence. Total excision of the mesorectum has, therefore, been carried out as a part of over 100 consecutive anterior resections. Fifty of these, which were classified as "curative" or "conceivably curative" operations, have now been followed for over 2 years with no pelvic or staple-line recurrence.

LS

This is the fundamental paper that has changed the approach to surgical management of rectal cancer and led to substantial improvements in the oncologic results of rectal cancer resection across the globe. The basis of this technique is the dissection of

© The Author(s), under exclusive license to Springer Nature Switzerland AG 2025
D. Colibaseanu et al., *Essential Articles in Colorectal Surgery*,
https://doi.org/10.1007/978-3-031-77745-5_8

the rectum surrounded by its mesorectum and enveloping fascia along the embryological planes separating it from the surrounding structures. This can accomplish both the removal of the perirectal lymph nodes at risk of loco-regional metastasis and the preservation of the pelvic autonomic nerves. The recommendation for this innovative surgical technique came together with the rejection of the once-common blunt dissection of the posterior rectum. It was postulated that violation of the mesorectal envelope by blunt dissection could lead to an increased risk of leaving tumor cells in the pelvis either through spillage or retention of portions of mesorectum. Under these circumstances, what is commonly referred to as local recurrence would be essentially a persistent tumor which would then regrow from the retained mesorectal tumor cells concentrically into the bowel and ultimately become endoscopically visible as recurrent cancer. The original paper recommended complete excision of the whole mesorectum in all cases of rectal cancer, but this was progressively amended to a tumor-specific mesorectal excision so that for more proximal lesions, a truly complete removal of the mesorectum with its inherent morbidity is not necessary [1]. The term total mesorectal excision (TME) has then evolved over time to indicate the principles of the technique which therefore also include cases of tumor-specific mesorectal excision. The adoption of the TME principles has resulted in a dramatic decrease in local recurrence rates after radical surgery for rectal cancer. These results have been repeated in different countries applying the same surgical technique as if replicating a successful scientific experiment [2]. A critical debate which stemmed from the publication of this and subsequent papers revolved on whether the impressive results of optimized surgery for rectal cancer would make it unnecessary to add neoadjuvant or adjuvant treatments. Historically, the impetus for their adoption had originated at least in part from the recognition of how dismal the rates of local recurrence used to be following surgery for rectal cancer. The evidence has indicated that the use of additional treatments following surgery performed using the TME principles does provide additional oncological benefits [3] so that in many cases, chemotherapy and radiotherapy should be viewed as complementary and not alternative to surgery. However, the debate persists on the appropriate indications for multimodality management as opposed to surgery alone. For example, upfront surgery without neoadjuvant chemoradiotherapy has been proposed for cT3 rectal lesions cephalad to 6 cm from the anal verge without threatened mesorectal fascia on pelvic magnetic resonance, regardless of any cN status [4]. At the opposite end of the spectrum is the approach referred to as watch-and-wait, in which total neoadjuvant treatment followed by complete clinical response could really become an alternative to surgery, in which the role of TME would be limited to salvage procedure in case of lesion regrowth.

References

1. Lopez-Kostner F, Lavery IC, Hool GR, Rybicki LA, Fazio VW. Total mesorectal excision is not necessary for cancers of the upper rectum. Surgery. 1998;124(4):612–7; discussion 617–8.
2. Knol J, Keller DS. Total mesorectal excision technique—past, present, and future. Clin Colon Rectal Surg. 2020;33(3):134–43.
3. Kapiteijn E, Marijnen CA, Nagtegaal ID, Putter H, Steup WH, Wiggers T, Rutten HJ, Pahlman L, Glimelius B, van Krieken JH, Leer JW, van de Velde CJ, Dutch Colorectal Cancer Group. Preoperative radiotherapy combined with total mesorectal excision for resectable rectal cancer. N Engl J Med. 2001;345(9):638–46.
4. Ruppert R, Junginger T, Kube R, Strassburg J, Lewin A, Baral J, Maurer CA, Sauer J, Lauscher J, Winde G, Thomasmeyer R, Stelzner S, Bambauer C, Scheunemann S, Faedrich A, Wollschlaeger D, Merkel S. Risk-adapted neoadjuvant chemoradiotherapy in rectal cancer: final report of the OCUM study. J Clin Oncol. 2023;41(24):4025–34.

Discussion

DC

This is another excellent series, and there is no doubt that it has changed rectal cancer surgery, becoming the gold standard for appropriate technique. Not many things last over four decades, yet this study remains just as relevant today. There are many controversial topics within the rectal cancer treatment world, but what constitutes an appropriate TME dissection is not one, and this was published before more than half of the readers were born.

LS

An aspect of this which I find impressive is that the description and subsequent adoption of a specific surgical technique went well beyond surgery and ultimately stimulated a corollary evolution in other specialties also treating rectal cancer. I am thinking of the surge of MR as the indispensable tool for locoregional staging, the changes in the assessment of the surgical specimen in pathology, and perhaps the subtler but still substantial changes in approaching the disease by medical and radiation oncology given the improvement in surgical outcomes, to the point that all specialists involved in rectal cancer care comfortably use the term "TME" in a tumor board discussion.

Similarity Between Sigmoid and High Rectal Cancers

9

Wilson SM, Beahrs OH. The curative treatment of carcinoma of the sigmoid, rectosigmoid, and rectum. Ann Surg. 1976;183(5):556–65.

Abstract

This retrospective series comprises 902 patients who underwent curative resection of the sigmoid colon, rectosigmoid, and upper rectum at the Mayo Clinic during the years 1959–1969. Lesions were divided according to the location from the dentate line, with 346 patients having had a lesion located more than 20 cm from the dentate line; in the remaining 556 patients, the lesion was between 6 and 20 cm distant. A thorough analysis was undertaken comparing these two groups of patients on the basis of operative mortality and morbidity, including anastomotic complications, 5- and 10-year survival, and incidence of local recurrence. Overall operative mortality was 1.9%, with an 8.1% incidence of anastomotic complications. The overall 5-year survival rate was 72% and the 10-year survival rate was 55%. The incidence of anastomotic recurrence for anastomosis performed with the use of extraperitoneal rectum was 5.8%; recurrence at the suture line developed in 2.9% of patients who underwent anastomosis to serosa-covered bowel. In addition to the above data, information will be presented which demonstrates the effect of the patient's height and weight on the surgeon's ability to perform a low-anterior anastomosis.

© The Author(s), under exclusive license to Springer Nature Switzerland AG 2025
D. Colibaseanu et al., *Essential Articles in Colorectal Surgery*,
https://doi.org/10.1007/978-3-031-77745-5_9

Finally, the incidence of anastomotic complications and of local recurrence was analyzed according to the intestinal preparation employed, the use of parenteral antibiotics, and the method of drainage used near the anastomosis.

LS

This series included over 900 patients undergoing restorative surgery for carcinoma of the sigmoid colon, rectosigmoid, and upper rectum between 1959 and 1969. Its analysis focused on a comparison of anterior resection and low anterior resection based on the hypothesis that since "the sigmoid, rectosigmoid and upper rectum shared a similar vascular and lymphatic supply" the "end result of resections of these areas might be the same." The term "anterior resection" referred to lesions in which the peritoneum was present both proximally and distally at the anastomosis, while "low anterior resection" was used when the distal end of the anastomosis was in the extraperitoneal rectum. All operations were performed transabdominally. There is no clear description of the operative technique, although it is mentioned that patients were treated with curative intent and only 38 out of 900 patients underwent creation of a diverting colostomy either at the time of their colorectal anastomosis or initially because of colonic obstruction. There is no mention of chemotherapy, radiotherapy, and especially surgical staplers, which had still to be introduced into practice. With all its limitations inevitably related to its time and the heterogeneity of the patient population, the results of these resections remain impressive, especially when we consider the absence of modern imaging. The 5-year local recurrence rates were 5.7% following anterior resection and 7.6% after low anterior resection. In this respect, the authors point out that a tumor distance of less than 8 cm from the anal verge was associated with increased risk of local recurrence, a finding which remains true to this day. The discussion of the paper advocates for anterior resection in the management of rectal cancer, which Claude Dixon, also at Mayo Clinic, had supported with the publication in 1948 of his own series of patients undergoing anterior resection, performed since 1930 as an alternative in selected cases to the systematic use of the abdominoperineal resection proposed by Miles [1]. It is also because of these early experiences and reports [2] that the debate on the oncologic appropriateness of anterior resection is long settled. The present paper did not emphasize particular aspects of the surgical technique but implies accurate patient selection and extraordinary mastery in the conduct of an oncologically radical rectal dissection. There is little doubt that the optimization of surgical technique is one of the main factors leading to a global improvement in oncologic results of rectal cancer treatment. A number of different institutions in the world have their own individual history leading to the progressive affirmation of modern surgery. More recently, William Heald and his seminal publication from 1982 introduced and popularized the concept of total mesorectal excision as the dissection of the rectum surrounded by its intact mesorectal fascia along embryological planes [3]. This is an oncologic principle which has remained ingrained in subsequent generations of surgeons as the multimodality management of rectal cancer has also evolved. This is an earlier and lesser-known publication which reveals an extraordinary tradition of excellence in surgical care, which precedes the concept of total mesorectal excision while likely applying its very principles.

References

1. Dixon CF. Anterior resection for malignant lesions of the upper part of the rectum and lower part of the sigmoid. Ann Surg. 1948;128(3):425–42.
2. Beahrs OH, Wilson SM. Cancer of the colon and rectum: a review of the newer technics in diagnosis and treatment. Adv Surg. 1975;9:235–46.
3. Heald RJ, Husband EM, Ryall RD. The mesorectum in rectal cancer surgery—the clue to pelvic recurrence? Br J Surg. 1982;69(10):613–6.

Discussion

DC

This study was published in 1976 and was the first of its kind. It is absolutely impressive. First, the meticulous recordkeeping for the era (this was 1959–1969), is absolutely astounding, and I've seen it myself, and have zero doubt that these 902 patients were able to be followed, a feat on its own. This was a high-volume center back then (and now), with almost 100 patients per year. The outcomes were excellent, and the surgical technique advanced and obviously meticulous. This was the "grand daddy" of TME.

LS

It is striking to see early data demonstrating concepts which are held true and current to this day. For example, the similarity between sigmoid and upper rectal cancer. While there was no discussion on adjuvant treatments in this paper, this hypothesis in retrospect resonates with the debate on avoiding radiotherapy in cases of upper rectal cancer, I am thinking for example at the PROSPECT trial. On the other hand, the data and comment on the increased aggressiveness and risk of local recurrence of rectal cancer originating in the distal 8 cm from the anal verge remind me of the current discussion on the indications for lateral pelvic lymph node dissection, which generally also pertains to distal rectal cancers.

Distance from the Anal Verge and Anastomotic Leak After Low Anterior Resection

10

Vignali A, Fazio VW, Lavery IC, Milsom JW, Church JM, Hull TL, Strong SA, Oakley JR. Factors associated with the occurrence of leaks in stapled rectal anastomoses: a review of 1014 patients. J Am Coll Surg. 1997;185(2):105–13.

Abstract

Background: Despite improvement in surgical techniques and stapling devices during the last 10 years, colorectal anastomoses are still prone to leakage. The purpose of this study was to assess the performance and safety of stapled anastomoses in rectal surgery and to identify factors that influence the occurrence of anastomotic leaks.

Study Design: A review of 1014 patients who underwent stapled anastomoses of the rectum or anal canal for colorectal cancer or benign disease between 1989 and 1995 in a tertiary care institution. Indications for operations, comorbidities at admission, preoperative bowel preparation, stapler size, intraoperative events, associated surgical procedures, and clinical outcomes were tested for any association with anastomotic leak.

Results: A double stapled technique was used in 154 patients and a conventional single stapler technique was used in 860. Postoperative mortality was 1.6%, and the overall morbidity was 18.4%. Clinically apparent anastomotic leak developed in 29 patients (2.9%). Anastomotic dehiscence occurred in 22 of 284 patients (7.7%) after low stapling (within 7 cm from the anal verge) and in 7 of 730 patients (1%) after high stapling ($p < 0.001$). Diabetes mellitus, use of pelvic drainage, and duration of surgery were significantly related to the occurrence of anastomotic leak by the univariate analysis. Multivariate regression analysis identified an anastomotic distance from the anal verge within 7 cm as the only variable related to the occurrence of postoperative leak ($p < 0.001$).

Conclusion: Low anastomoses were associated with a leak rate greater than with high colorectal anastomoses. We conclude that anastomoses to the rectum using the circular stapler can be done with low mortality and morbidity.

LS

This is the classical paper on stapled colorectal anastomosis and the association between distance of the anastomosis from the anal verge and risk of anastomotic failure. The authors retrospectively analyzed 1014 patients who underwent stapled colorectal anastomosis for either cancer or a variety of benign diseases. The anastomotic distance from the anal verge was divided into 3–7 cm, 8–11 cm, or greater than 11 cm. The anastomotic technique (single stapled vs. double stapled), the size of the stapler used, and the decision to place a pelvic drain or to create an additional fecal diversion were left at the discretion of the operating surgeon. A clinically apparent anastomotic leak developed in 29 patients (2.9%). The anastomotic leak rate for a distance from the anastomosis of 3–7 cm was 7.8%, while the leak rates for the 8–11 cm range and for anastomoses higher than 11 cm from the anal verge were 1% for each group. A number of patient-related, disease-related, and treatment-related variables were assessed for possible association with anastomotic leak. On univariate analysis, insulin-dependent diabetes mellitus and placement of a pelvic drain were significantly associated with an anastomotic leak ($p = 0.039$ and 0.018, respectively), unlike the technique of stapling, size of the stapler, or fecal diversion. The only factor which remained significantly associated with anastomotic leak both on univariate and on multivariate analysis was a shorter anastomotic distance from the anal verge ($p = 0.001$ and $p < 0.001$, respectively). Based on this study, many surgeons including me favor stoma diversion for all colorectal anastomoses within the distal 7 cm from the anal verge, regardless of previous radiotherapy or other risk factors. I realize it is possible to be more selective and that ileostomy management and ileostomy closure are associated with their own morbidity. However, a stoma diversion, typically an ileostomy in my case, at least reduces the degree of morbidity should an anastomotic leak occur. An anastomotic leak following an undiverted low colorectal or coloanal anastomosis easily leads to permanent colostomy. It is true that diffuse peritonitis after diverting ileostomy closure can be a challenging situation, especially in a high-risk patient, but this complication does not lead to permanent colostomy. This study carries inevitable limitations. Most of the anastomoses in the analysis were created using the single-stapled technique, while most of us prefer the double-stapled technique, which both in the present and in many other subsequent studies has not been associated with an increased risk of anastomotic failure. Some important variables such as preoperative use of radiation therapy or steroid use were not significant factors in the analysis but seemed underpowered to provide reliable data. Importantly, the study population is obviously limited to open surgery and does not provide information on colorectal anastomoses performed using minimally invasive techniques. A recent review examining 25 studies indicated a median anastomotic leak rate of 7.3%, ranging from 0.7% to 24.5%. The most commonly reported predictors of anastomotic leak after the double-stapled technique were low tumor location, multiple stapler firings, male sex, longer operation time, and perioperative blood transfusion [1]. While there is still debate on the relationship between multiple staple firings for rectal transection and colorectal or coloanal anastomotic leak, all other variables are widely accepted as risk factors, although they were not clearly identified in the present article. Despite its limitation, this work establishes a useful, practical guideline based on clear numbers to inform a surgeon's decision on when to create a stoma diversion in addition to low anterior resection.

Reference

1. Emile SH, Barsom SH, Elfallal AH, Wexner SD. Comprehensive literature review of the outcome, modifications, and alternatives to double-stapled low pelvic colorectal anastomosis. Surgery. 2022;172(2):512–21.

Discussion

DC

My comments on this article are similar to the Mathiessen article (Chap. 17). The distance from the anal verge of a potential anastomosis is a marker for multiple factors that increase the risk of a leak, which are surgery-specific factors (tension, blood supply, how much distal bowel is left), patient factors (immunosuppression, general health), and what a leak would entail for the specific patient in question. I might not divert if the patient has no history of radiotherapy, the anastomosis had no tension, and there was good blood supply.

MD

What is your cutoff?

DC

Well, there are patients where the colon does not reach well, or the operation is just more difficult.

MD

This paper nicely demonstrates risk factors associated with the anastomotic leak, particularly with regard to the level of the anastomosis. Being trained at Cleveland Clinic, this was always a guide for when to divert patients undergoing low anterior resection, and I continue to use this in my practice today. Dr. Colibaseanu mentioned that for him, regardless of the height of the anastomosis, he is comfortable with a primary anastomosis and not diverting if there is no tension, adequate blood supply, and optimal patient characteristics (no immunosuppression, not malnourished, etc.). Diverting loop ileostomy comes with its significant potential complications, particularly dehydration, electrolyte abnormalities, and acute renal failure.

In my opinion, the risk of long-term consequences of an anastomotic leak and pelvic sepsis with a low pelvic anastomosis (less than 5 cm) that could result in a permanent stoma or significant functional compromise outweighs the benefits of avoiding fecal diversion in these cases. Though patients may suffer short-term complications from a diverting loop ileostomy, this fecal diversion may ultimately aid in salvaging their rectum or preserving anorectal function should an anastomotic leak occur. While again it is not just a strict cutoff, even in a healthy individual who may have no other medical issues and an anastomosis at 4–5 cm, even when everything looks great. I am more liberal in diverting. More so because at the same time, I would not want my young, healthy patient to leak and then end up needing a permanent stoma or having very poor function because of an undiverted leak.

The main drawbacks I find in this study that do not apply to my practice are the primary use of a single-stapled technique and open surgery. That being said, the quality of surgery reported in this large study from a high-volume institution speaks to the validity of their findings, and so I continue to use a 7 cm cutoff for when to consider fecal diversion in patients undergoing low anterior resection.

AM

I think similarly to the comments we had on other papers. To me, it is never really a height number because the measurement from the anal verge can be very variable, as everyone's kind of stated, and we have all encountered that, and everyone's anuses are a little bit of a different length. Just picking a cutoff to me does not really make much sense, and it is instead a number of factors we put back together to make a judgment regarding whether we think the risk of diversion is lower than the risk of a leak.

LS

This is an old article that presents evidence supporting the idea of different risks based on the distance of the anastomosis from the anal verge, although I recognize that the decision to add a stoma diversion remains multifactorial. As we are discussing this article, I feel we go through themes which recur in the discussion of other articles about anastomotic leak risk factors or when we should divert. I agree that these were all open cases, and a single-stapled technique was used in the majority of patients, which might not relate to many contemporary cases.

DC

From my perspective, there are very specific factors that are associated with a higher leak rate in lower anastomosis. Those are very practical ones. Reach (and therefore tension) is almost always the primary culprit here. A mid rectal anastomosis with no tension, in an otherwise unremarkable operation, in a healthy patient should have a very low risk of a leak. I do not think there is anything mysterious at all about how low an anastomosis exists; as long as the blood supply is great, there is no tension on the anastomosis in an otherwise technically adequate surgery.

You make the point of focusing on what to do if they leak. If I can reach the anastomosis and over-sew it, I think about not diverting, but obviously all the other factors I've mentioned above need to be considered.

I concede the point to Michelle that a low anastomotic leak without diversion is very difficult to rescue if a permanent stoma is to be avoided.

The Fundamental Role of Magnetic Resonance in Rectal Cancer Staging

11

MERCURY Study Group. Diagnostic accuracy of preoperative magnetic resonance imaging in predicting curative resection of rectal cancer: prospective observational study. BMJ. 2006;333(7572):779.

Abstract

Objective: To assess the accuracy of preoperative staging of rectal cancer with magnetic resonance imaging to predict surgical circumferential resection margins.

Design: Prospective observational study of rectal cancers treated by colorectal multidisciplinary teams between January 2002 and October 2003.

Setting: 11 colorectal units in four European countries.

Participants: 408 consecutive patients presenting with all stages of rectal cancer and undergoing magnetic resonance imaging before total mesorectal excision surgery and histopathological assessment of the surgical specimen.

Main outcome measures: Accuracy of magnetic resonance imaging in predicting a curative resection based on the histological yardstick of presence or absence of tumor at the margins of the specimen.

Results: 354 of the 408 patients had a clear circumferential resection margin (87%, 95% confidence interval 83–90%). Specificity for prediction of a clear margin by magnetic resonance

© The Author(s), under exclusive license to Springer Nature Switzerland AG 2025
D. Colibaseanu et al., *Essential Articles in Colorectal Surgery*, https://doi.org/10.1007/978-3-031-77745-5_11

imaging was 92% (327/354, 90–95%). High-resolution scans were technically satisfactory in 93% (379/408). Surgical specimens were histopathologically graded as complete or moderate in 80% (328/408), and the median lymph node harvest was 12 (range 0–49). Magnetic resonance imaging predicted clear margins in 349 patients. At surgery, 327 had clear margins (94%, 91–96%).

Conclusion: High-resolution magnetic resonance imaging accurately predicts whether the surgical resection margins will be clear or affected by tumor. This technique can be reproduced accurately in multiple centers to predict curative resection and warns the multidisciplinary team of potential failure of surgery, thus enabling selection of patients for preoperative treatment.

DC

This was a prospective observational study originating from 11 hospitals in 4 European countries. The primary objective of this study was to assess the accuracy of Magnetic Resonance Imaging (MRI) to predict negative surgical resection margins. This study enrolled 408 patients from January 2002 to October 2003.

In addition to MRI evaluation by the 18 radiologists (5–20 years experience in abdominal MRI) who underwent workshops in preparation for this study, 30 colorectal surgeons evaluated the tumors with a digital rectal examination and flexible sigmoidoscopy. All patients were discussed preoperatively at multidisciplinary tumor team meetings. For patients with threatened margins, they had either extended resections, radiation, or chemoradiation prior to surgery. All pathologists were experienced GI histopathologists who underwent specialized workshops to prepare for this study.

Ultimately, in patients who went straight to surgery (i.e., they were predicted to have a negative margin), the accuracy of predicting a clear margin was 91% with a negative predictive value of 97%. In those who had received radiation or chemoradiation therapy, the accuracy was 77% with a negative predictive value of 98%.

The difficulty with the MRI was in distinguishing those patients who had tumor or treatment scarring at the margin, overcalling tumor even in cases where there was treatment effect but no residual tumor.

I think that this was a pivotal study in the treatment of rectal cancer. Prior to this point—and the results of this did not trickle down for a few years—it seemed that staging could be assessed with either endorectal ultrasound or MRI; now, nearly universally, I will obtain an MRI. The only addition (and not exception) would be adding EUS for a case where MRI cannot distinguish between a T1 and T2, and I am considering a transanal approach, or if there is a node in a T1 tumor that looks suspicious and is accessible transanally.

So, from my perspective, the proverbial horse is out of the barn. I do not see us ever not using MRI as the primary modality for local staging of rectal cancer. In fact, multiple (and I lost count of how many) MERCURY babies (f/u studies) have proven the utility of MRI by showing that the depth of extramural tumor is also predictable [1], and MRI is also very good for determining circumferential margin and distal margin in post chemoradiation treatment [2]. So, I think the matter is settled for me. Maybe the second biggest advance since total mesorectal excision (TME).

References

1. MERCURY Study Group. Extramural depth of tumor invasion at thin-section MR in patients with rectal cancer: results of MERCURY study. Radiology. 2007;43(1):132–9.
2. Patel UB, et al. MRI after treatment of locally advanced rectal cancer: how to report tumor response—the MERCURY experience. AJR. 2012;199:486–95.

Discussion

DC

If I do not have an MRI ready for a case presentation at the tumor board, I will have to relist the case until I get the MRI. It is very rare that we could even think of a situation where we would not use MRI.

MD

Yes, I completely agree; this study marked a pivotal change in how we approach the staging of rectal cancer, to the extent that it's now integrated into the NCCN guidelines, advocating MRI as the preferred imaging tool. It's remarkable that the study compared MRI to a digital rectal exam, a comparison almost unfathomable today. Regardless, the study effectively supplanted ultrasound in our staging protocols, except in the smaller T1 and T2 lesions where ultrasound has improved accuracy.

Now, we have to remember, this study was published in 2006… Fast forward to today, in the era of total neoadjuvant therapy (TNT), where nonoperative management and a watch-and-wait approach are increasingly utilized and often preferred. Now, the conversation surrounding MRIs revolves around staging tumors or predicting a complete clinical response, post-neoadjuvant chemoradiation, and TNT which differs significantly from its accuracy in staging untreated tumors, as evidenced by newer literature. Though the accuracy of ultrasound is notoriously operator-dependent, there is also significant variability in MRI which is dependent on factors like machine quality, software, and technique.

LS

I agree, it is impressive how this study still defines the management of rectal cancer over 20 years after the enrollment of the original study patients. Reading that the accuracy of the MR was compared to digital rectal examination speaks to how revolutionary this study was. Our weekly tumor board discussions on neoadjuvant treatment and surgery for rectal cancer remain centered around MR images. In addition, the role of MR is critical when deciding on pelvic lymphadenectomy or intraoperative radiotherapy. One aspect that is also problematic to me is to note a persistent difference in quality among MRs performed in different institutions, despite the original impetus to establish workshops for radiologists, for which the original authors of this multicenter study advocated. At the same time, similar workshops involved pathologists and, of course, surgeons, to standardize rectal cancer management. I feel that rectal cancer treatment in general is better today than it was 20 years ago, and part of the credit for it should go to the MERCURY trial. However, I wish that the quality of MR pelvis to stage rectal cancer was as consistent as a CT chest, abdomen, and pelvis, for example.

I admire those who designed this trial because I think that conceiving MR as a staging modality comes along with conceiving circumferential radial margin as the critical regional staging measurement, and I think that our oncologists feel the same. However, circumferential radial margin is not the only factor, because I think that lymph node involvement in the mesorectum is an independent factor associated with risk of recurrence. The other issue that has been investigated through the MR images is the involvement of the pelvic lymph nodes, and MR remains suboptimal in assessing lymph nodes. So, there is still a subset of patients who have silent, invisible involvement of pelvic lymph nodes, and they ultimately recur because of that.

Preoperative vs. Postoperative Chemoradiotherapy for Rectal Cancer

12

Sauer R, Becker H, Hohenberger W, et al., German Rectal Cancer Study Group. Preoperative versus postoperative chemoradiotherapy for rectal cancer. N Engl J Med. 2004;351(17):1731–40.

Abstract

Background: Postoperative chemoradiotherapy is the recommended standard therapy for patients with locally advanced rectal cancer. In recent years, encouraging results with preoperative radiotherapy have been reported. We compared preoperative chemoradiotherapy with postoperative chemoradiotherapy for locally advanced rectal cancer.

Methods: We randomly assigned patients with clinical stage T3 or T4 or node-positive disease to receive either preoperative or postoperative chemoradiotherapy. The preoperative treatment consisted of 5040 cGy delivered in fractions of 180 cGy per day, 5 days per week, and fluorouracil, given in a 120-h continuous intravenous infusion at a dose of 1000 mg per square meter of body-surface area per day during the first and fifth weeks of radiotherapy. Surgery was performed 6 weeks after the completion of chemoradiotherapy. One month after surgery, four 5-day cycles of fluorouracil (500 mg per square meter per day) were given. Chemoradiotherapy was identical in the postoperative-treatment group, except for the delivery of a boost of 540 cGy. The primary endpoint was overall survival.

© The Author(s), under exclusive license to Springer Nature Switzerland AG 2025

73

D. Colibaseanu et al., *Essential Articles in Colorectal Surgery*,
https://doi.org/10.1007/978-3-031-77745-5_12

Results: Four hundred twenty-one patients were randomly assigned to receive preoperative chemoradiotherapy and 402 patients to receive postoperative chemoradiotherapy. The overall 5-year survival rates were 76% and 74%, respectively ($P = 0.80$). The 5-year cumulative incidence of local relapse was 6% for patients assigned to preoperative chemoradiotherapy and 13% in the postoperative-treatment group ($P = 0.006$). Grade 3 or 4 acute toxic effects occurred in 27% of the patients in the preoperative-treatment group, as compared with 40% of the patients in the postoperative-treatment group ($P = 0.001$); the corresponding rates of long-term toxic effects were 14% and 24%, respectively ($P = 0.01$).

Conclusions: Preoperative chemoradiotherapy, as compared with postoperative chemoradiotherapy, improved local control and was associated with reduced toxicity but did not improve overall survival.

LS

This trial determined a fundamental shift in practice at least in the United States and solidified the role of preoperative chemoradiotherapy in the treatment of stage II–III rectal cancer. Its results indicated a significant reduction in treatment-related toxicity in favor of long-course preoperative chemoradiotherapy, and this is perhaps the main reason this modality has been widely preferred since. However, the result of the analysis also emphasized some known limitations of preoperative treatments. Eighteen percent of patients who were randomized to the postoperative chemoradiotherapy arm were found to have stage I cancer on their surgical specimen and were therefore overstaged. Because of their pathology staging, they never received chemoradiotherapy and therefore were never subject to its inherent risks. Given the randomization design, we could reasonably estimate that a similar proportion of patients in the preoperative chemoradiotherapy arm were actually overtreated. Therefore, the reported reduction in local recurrence rate associated with neoadjuvant chemoradiotherapy could be caused at least in part by overstaging rather than a truly increased effectiveness of preoperative treatment on the patient's native, well-perfused tissues. Patients enrolled in the trial were staged using endorectal ultrasound and Computed Tomography scan, and it is possible that with modern Magnetic Resonance of the pelvis, the risk of overstaging is reduced. However, I still feel that the statement that preoperative chemoradiotherapy is associated with a reduction in local recurrence rate should be made with caution. Another important principle associated with this work is that 39% of patients in the preoperative treatment arm for whom an abdominoperineal resection was deemed necessary at the time of their preoperative evaluation could have a sphincter-preserving surgery after neoadjuvant chemoradiotherapy. This challenges the clinical practice of several surgeons who decide on sphincter preservation before initiation of any neoadjuvant treatments. The idea behind this tradition is the belief that some viable tumor cells could still be left in place in areas where the tumor is no longer visible after neoadjuvant treatment. This trial provides compelling evidence against this assumption and informs current clinical practice to this day. The results after a median follow-up of 11 years following the original trial corroborate the idea of deciding on sphincter preservation only after neoadjuvant treatment has been completed. The updated trial results indicate once more a reduced local recurrence rate associated with the preoperative arm without any differences in overall survival, disease-free survival, or cumulative incidence of distant metastasis [1]. In retrospect, this trial and the widespread acceptance of preoperative chemoradiotherapy ended up creating the foundations for the increasing use of total neoadjuvant therapy (TNT) [2], and the very principle of deciding on surgery based on the results of the initial treatment received is what made organ preservation conceivable. The current guidelines still recommend postoperative chemoradiotherapy for patients who have stage II or III rectal cancer on pathology and have not received preoperative treatments [3]. However, it has become rare to discuss postoperative chemoradiotherapy for rectal cancer at our tumor board, which is probably to the benefit of our patients.

References

1. Sauer R, Liersch T, Merkel S, Fietkau R, Hohenberger W, Hess C, Becker H, Raab HR, Villanueva MT, Witzigmann H, Wittekind C, Beissbarth T, Rödel C. Preoperative versus postoperative chemoradiotherapy for locally advanced rectal cancer: results of the German CAO/ARO/AIO-94 randomized phase III trial after a median follow-up of 11 years. J Clin Oncol. 2012;30(16):1926–33.
2. Liu J, Ladbury C, Glaser S, Fakih M, Kaiser AM, Chen YJ, Williams TM, Amini A. Patterns of care for patients with locally advanced rectal cancer treated with total neoadjuvant therapy at predominately academic centers between 2016–2020: an NCDB analysis. Clin Colorectal Cancer. 2023;22(2):167–74.
3. Benson AB, Venook AP, Al-Hawary MM, Azad N, Chen YJ, Ciombor KK, Cohen S, Cooper HS, Deming D, Garrido-Laguna I, Grem JL, Gunn A, Hecht JR, Hoffe S, Hubbard J, Hunt S, Jeck W, Johung KL, Kirilcuk N, Krishnamurthi S, Maratt JK, Messersmith WA, Meyerhardt J, Miller ED, Mulcahy MF, Nurkin S, Overman MJ, Parikh A, Patel H, Pedersen K, Saltz L, Schneider C, Shibata D, Skibber JM, Sofocleous CT, Stotsky-Himelfarb E, Tavakkoli A, Willett CG, Gregory K, Gurski L. Rectal cancer, version 2.2022, NCCN Clinical Practice Guidelines in Oncology. J Natl Compr Canc Netw. 2022;20(10):1139–67.

Discussion

MD

I think that this paper definitely revolutionized the way how we treat rectal cancer. I agree with the nuance on overstaging which is usually not emphasized as much. Most people do talk about preoperative radiotherapy as associated with decreased local recurrence rates because of this study besides decreased toxicity rates compared to postoperative therapy.

With respect to deciding on sphincter preservation, I remember when I was training at Cleveland Clinic, certainly, the teaching was that the need for an APR was determined by the pretreatment MRI, despite the findings of this study, which were published many years prior to me being there. And I agree on that with regard to watch-and-wait.

Now that it has become evident that this is an appropriate treatment strategy, we have to accept that operative planning can be made after neoadjuvant therapy. So, the principle of deciding before initiation of treatment is hard for me to accept.

DC

At least for me, at the beginning of my career, the decision on the operative approach was being made on pretreatment imaging and clinical findings. Interval imaging (between chemoradiation and surgery) did not change the level of transection or the operation performed. Though this trial's intent was not to look at TNT (total neoadjuvant therapy), I think that we would find the seeds of that idea here. And so, in many ways, it is a crucial trial.

There are a lot of theories with regard to tumor regression, whether the tumor dies off or regresses in a mosaic pattern or linear pattern, and so forth. There were a lot of theories regarding whether the transection level should be affected by the regression of tumor that oftentimes we see with chemoradiotherapy. I think that those questions still linger today, many years after the trial.

The cat is out of the bag, so to speak, with regards to utilization of chemoradiotherapy, and I think that has expanded; and now, I anticipate we will do fewer surgeries on patients that have TNT, for example, and though this is obviously not TNT, to me, it is the seed that germinated into TNT.

AM

I think it is not really debated at all anymore whether we should use neoadjuvant vs. adjuvant chemoradiotherapy, but I think even at the time when the German rectal cancer trial was published, as you stated, this concept of shifting decision for surgery based on response was still debated and even in the era of the training paradigms that have been discussed, I think. There was still variability, but at least I think it sounds like in our respective institutions probably, surgeons tended more toward the pretreatment decision. This was carried forward regardless of tumor response. But I do not think that is really as strongly debated now, and it is far more accepted that your treatment potentially changes based on results. Maybe it is a little bit risky to say, but maybe, that is actually the more interesting finding of the German trial. But I think there is other evidence to support that despite data suggesting what you were mentioning with respect to the mosaic distribution of response, there are also other data, definitely other data to support change in treatment decision based on tumor response.

LS

Do you feel that at Mayo, for example, in the years 2005–2010 or so, this issue of deciding on sphincter preservation before treatment was the existing culture? Or was it pretty much accepted that after treatment, if the patient responded well, sphincters could be preserved as a result of shrinking of the primary tumors? The vast majority would make that decision based on preoperative imaging, and it would not change. So that is I guess what we would call the general practice at that time.

DC

Yes, and that is what I was saying earlier that the level of transection, at least for me, had always been made pretreatment based on the imaging and clinical findings of pre-chemoradiotherapy rather than post-chemoradiotherapy. And even if the tumor regressed, many still did not change the transection level.

Synergy Between Preoperative Radiotherapy and Surgery in the Treatment of Rectal Cancer

13

Kapiteijn E, Marijnen CA, Nagtegaal ID, Putter H, Steup WH, Wiggers T, Rutten HJ, Pahlman L, Glimelius B, van Krieken JH, Leer JW, van de Velde CJ; Dutch Colorectal Cancer Group. Preoperative radiotherapy combined with total mesorectal excision for resectable rectal cancer. N Engl J Med. 2001;345(9):638–46.

Abstract

Background: Short-term preoperative radiotherapy followed by total mesorectal excision has been shown to improve local control of disease in patients with resectable rectal cancer. We conducted a multicenter, randomized trial to determine whether the addition of preoperative radiotherapy increases the benefit of total mesorectal excision.

Methods: We randomly assigned 1861 patients with resectable rectal cancer either to preoperative radiotherapy (5 Gy on each of 5 days) followed by total mesorectal excision (924 patients) or to total mesorectal excision alone (937 patients). The trial was conducted with the use of standardization and quality control measures to ensure the consistency of the radiotherapy, surgery, and pathological techniques.

Results: Of the 1861 patients randomly assigned to one of the two treatment groups, 1805 were eligible to participate. The overall rate of survival at 2 years among the eligible patients was

© The Author(s), under exclusive license to Springer Nature
Switzerland AG 2025
D. Colibaseanu et al., *Essential Articles in Colorectal Surgery*,
https://doi.org/10.1007/978-3-031-77745-5_13

82.0% in the group assigned to both radiotherapy and surgery and 81.8% in the group assigned to surgery alone ($P = 0.84$). Among the 1748 patients who underwent a macroscopically complete local resection, the rate of local recurrence at 2 years was 5.3%. The rate of local recurrence at 2 years was 2.4% in the radiotherapy-plus-surgery group and 8.2% in the surgery-only group ($P < 0.001$).

Conclusions: Short-term preoperative radiotherapy reduces the risk of local recurrence in patients with rectal cancer who undergo a standardized total mesorectal excision.

LS

The Dutch trial has contributed to establish the role of neoadjuvant radiotherapy as complementary and not alternative to optimized radical surgery for rectal cancer in minimizing the risk of local recurrence rate. This was the first large multicenter prospective randomized trial where the use of radiotherapy was evaluated in a large group of patients in whom surgery for rectal cancer was meticulously standardized through workshops and other educational materials to perform an adequate total mesorectal excision. The successful use of short-course preoperative radiotherapy in combination with total mesorectal excision was also the base for subsequent trials. After a median follow-up of 24.9 months, patients receiving neoadjuvant radiotherapy before surgery were associated with a significantly reduced local recurrence rate, 2.4% vs. 8.2% following surgery alone. Overall survival was similar. Long-term results after a median 11.6-year follow-up among surviving patients confirmed a reduced 10-year cumulative incidence of local recurrence, which was 5% in the radiotherapy group vs. 11% in the surgery-alone group. Out of all individuals experiencing local recurrence, the proportion presenting later than 5 years after surgery was 11% in the surgery-alone group and 9% in the irradiated group. There were again no differences between groups in overall survival. The reduction in mortality for rectal cancer in the irradiated group was offset by an increased death rate from other causes, which included secondary malignancy. On the other hand, in the subgroup of patients with stage III cancer and negative circumferential resection margin on pathology, the use of preoperative short-course radiotherapy was associated with a significant 10-year survival advantage [1]. This indicates that radiotherapy can be beneficial but is also associated with substantial long-term risks, and its use should be focused on those disease presentations at elevated risk of local recurrence. The debate on the exact boundaries of this patient subgroup remains open. In this respect, patients enrolled in the Dutch trial did not have their tumors staged using modern pelvic MR imaging, which can lead today to a better patient selection. Individuals with all rectal cancer stages were randomized, including those with stage I disease. This resulted in overtreatment in a substantial proportion of patients. The preparation and design of the Dutch trial were possible through extraordinary and unprecedented efforts. The low local recurrence rates, particularly in the study group, speak to the advancements in the management of rectal cancer. Despite compelling evidence from this and other well-designed trials, neoadjuvant short-course radiotherapy remains rarely utilized in the United States. While this might be based on individual preferences and strictly medical decision-making, it also at least in part depends on reimbursement disadvantages associated with short-course radiotherapy when compared to the more frequently used long-course radiotherapy [2].

References

1. van Gijn W, Marijnen CA, Nagtegaal ID, Kranenbarg EM, Putter H, Wiggers T, Rutten HJ, Påhlman L, Glimelius B, van de Velde CJ; Dutch Colorectal Cancer Group. Preoperative radiotherapy combined with total mesorectal excision for resectable rectal cancer: 12-year follow-up of the multicentre, randomised controlled TME trial. Lancet Oncol. 2011;12(6):575–82.
2. Mowery YM, Salama JK, Zafar SY, Moore HG, Willett CG, Czito BG, Hopkins MB, Palta M. Neoadjuvant long-course chemoradiation remains strongly favored over short-course radiotherapy by radiation oncologists in the United States. Cancer. 2017;123(8):1434–1441.

Discussion

MD

One striking aspect of this study was that when looking at the height of the tumor, the investigators found benefit with regard to local recurrence in tumors located at less than 10 cm from the anal verge. The use of radiotherapy for upper rectal tumors is more controversial, and here, we generally do not radiate them, but this clearly showed there was not any benefit from radiation therapy in the upper rectal tumors. Do you know why they decided to use short course in this study instead of traditionally long course?

LS

I think it is more of their traditional practice. Apart from any discussion on indications, I have to recognize that short-course treatment is at least more convenient. I mean, if I were a patient and somebody tells me I can receive radiotherapy for a week and, the following Monday or Tuesday, I can have surgery for rectal cancer, a condition which makes me upset and distraught, I would prefer it in terms of practicality. And I think that it is also important to point out that there is some data indicating that the decision to give long course or short course, at least in part, is related to reimbursement [2] with long-course treatment being associated with better reimbursement. So, if you put this kind of decision-making within a fragmented healthcare environment where the majority of physicians are private practitioners, this does matter. For example, if you are at Washington University in St. Louis receiving a salary, you can promote short-course treatment which they have historically investigated and used in the United States with good science and good data. But if you are a private practitioner, I think it is difficult to promote something when there is some debate about the fractionation and risk of increased toxicity associated with short course, and on top of that, you know that you will be paid less. Unless you feel strongly from a scientific standpoint, what would be the incentive to give short course ther-

apy to your patients? I think that this is an important part of the
debate on why we do not use this more in the United States.

AM

I think you are definitely right. When you look at the penetrance
of short-course radiotherapy throughout Europe, it is to a far
greater degree than in the United States. I think those economic
factors definitely play a role.

DC

I find this study very impressive. Here we are 23 years later, and
we are still talking about the study and its results. It is very rare to
see a study like this where it is quoted even now, and we talk about
this study not infrequently in our tumor board. So, I think the
work that they did is outstanding. Having said that, I do not want
to say shortcomings, but there are limitations to what we can
interpret from the study. The authors could probably tell us a lot
more clearly on what their exact intent was, but I think that their
data indicate that using radiation in appropriate patients reduces
the local recurrence rate by half. That is an easy figure to remember and something I still talk to my patients about, so I think it is
a great study. I agree with the comments on short-course variability with regard to its implementation. I think that the question of
whether short course versus long course has better or worse oncologic outcomes and better or worse side effects for patients is the
question that we might clearly identify and then choose, but I
think that the scale is probably tipped toward short-course radiation, it is just a matter of implementation.

AM

I think the thing that goes hand in hand with deciding short course
vs. long course, which has been seen in more recent trials, has

been the timing of surgery, which is still undefined and still debated even in the setting of long-course chemoradiotherapy. And speaking of at least more contemporary studies, long-term results in the RAPIDO trial have shown an increased loco-regional recurrence rate for those patients who had a delay to surgery after short-course radiotherapy.

LS

I agree, and I think that the other issue that has come to the fore is that there is no organized school of thought advocating through publications short course radiotherapy within the context of non-operative management of rectal cancer. That, to me, will impair the potential popularity of short course. We will discuss RAPIDO separately, but it is obvious that RAPIDO, unlike OPRA, was never intended to select a group of patients who will continue with nonoperative management.

DC

Let us say that you only had one choice, either long term or short term to use a radiotherapy modality to all your patients. Which one would you use? Long course? *(after hearing feedback from others)* Long course. All right.

Avoiding Radiotherapy in Selected Cases of Rectal Cancer

14

Schrag D, Shi Q, Weiser MR, Gollub MJ, Saltz LB, Musher BL, Goldberg J, Al Baghdadi T, Goodman KA, McWilliams RR, Farma JM, George TJ, Kennecke HF, Shergill A, Montemurro M, Nelson GD, Colgrove B, Gordon V, Venook AP, O'Reilly EM, Meyerhardt JA, Dueck AC, Basch E, Chang GJ, Mamon HJ. Preoperative treatment of locally advanced rectal cancer. N Engl J Med. 2023;389(4):322–334.

Abstract

Background: Pelvic radiation plus sensitizing chemotherapy with a fluoropyrimidine (chemoradiotherapy) before surgery is standard care for locally advanced rectal cancer in North America. Whether neoadjuvant chemotherapy with fluorouracil, leucovorin, and oxaliplatin (FOLFOX) can be used in lieu of chemoradiotherapy is uncertain.

Methods: We conducted a multicenter, unblinded, noninferiority, randomized trial of neoadjuvant FOLFOX (with chemoradiotherapy given only if the primary tumor decreased in size by <20% or if FOLFOX was discontinued because of side effects) as compared with chemoradiotherapy. Adults with rectal cancer that had been clinically staged as T2 node-positive, T3 node-negative, or T3 node-positive who were candidates for sphincter-sparing surgery were eligible to participate. The primary endpoint was disease-free survival. Noninferiority would be claimed if the upper limit of the two-sided 90.2% confidence interval of the hazard ratio for disease recurrence or death did not exceed 1.29. Secondary endpoints included overall survival, local recurrence (in a time-to-event analysis), complete pathological resection, complete response, and toxic effects.

Results: From June 2012 through December 2018, a total of 1194 patients underwent randomization and 1128 started treatment; among those who started treatment, 585 were in the FOLFOX group and 543 in the chemoradiotherapy group. At a median follow-up of 58 months, FOLFOX was noninferior to chemoradiotherapy for disease-free survival (hazard ratio for disease recurrence or death, 0.92; 90.2% confidence interval [CI], 0.74–1.14; $P = 0.005$ for noninferiority). Five-year disease-free survival was 80.8% (95% CI, 77.9–83.7) in the FOLFOX group and 78.6% (95% CI, 75.4–81.8) in the chemoradiotherapy group. The groups were similar with respect to overall survival (hazard ratio for death, 1.04; 95% CI, 0.74–1.44) and local recurrence (hazard ratio, 1.18; 95% CI, 0.44–3.16). In the FOLFOX group, 53 patients (9.1%) received preoperative chemoradiotherapy and 8 (1.4%) received postoperative chemoradiotherapy.

Conclusions: In patients with locally advanced rectal cancer who were eligible for sphincter-sparing surgery, preoperative FOLFOX was noninferior to preoperative chemoradiotherapy with respect to disease-free survival.

LS

This trial compared neoadjuvant FOLFOX and traditional long-course chemoradiotherapy in patients with rectal cancer candidates for sphincter sparing surgery and clinically staged as T2–3 N+ or T3N0. In the experimental FOLFOX group, patients who did not achieve at least a 20% decrease in tumor size after FOLFOX treatment or discontinued FOLFOX because of side effects received chemoradiotherapy and remained in the FOLFOX group in an intent-to-treat analysis. The PROSPECT trial is unique in its focus on what could be defined as intermediate-risk patients who are expected to have a restorative procedure. This inherently excludes some of the most difficult rectal cancer cases and those at highest risk of recurrence. After a median follow-up of 58 months, the study groups were comparable with a 5-year disease-free survival of 80.8% versus 78.6% in the FOLFOX and chemoradiotherapy groups, respectively. The percentage of patients initially assigned to the FOLFOX group who ended up receiving preoperative chemoradiotherapy was 9.1%, while 1.4% received postoperative chemoradiotherapy. The strategy of upfront chemotherapy alone was therefore successful in this particular patient population, and the results support the decision to avoid radiotherapy in this patient group with its associated side effects. This trial took a long time to accrue, from June 2012 through December 2018. At the time of its publication in 2023, one could argue that the standard of care of long-course chemoradiotherapy is at least being challenged by total neoadjuvant therapy (TNT). However, this analysis supports avoiding radiotherapy at least in a subgroup of patients with higher rectal cancers having in general a decreased risk of local recurrence. This approach is useful to me as a practicing surgeon for cancers that are straddling the peritoneal reflection, which has generated endless debates at our tumor board on whether they should be treated as sigmoid cancer or rectal cancer. We have contemporary data on the safety and effectiveness of neoadjuvant chemotherapy for locally advanced colon cancer [1] plus the results of this trial to corroborate the use of neoadjuvant chemotherapy in these patients. This should therefore obviate at least in the majority of cases the question on how to label a rectosigmoid lesion. The other potential advantage coming from PROSPECT is that traditionally patients with neoadjuvant long-course chemoradiotherapy have undergone stoma diversion at the time of their anterior resection, and perhaps, this could be spared in a larger proportion of patients receiving only chemotherapy before surgery. This will require further studies. This trial implies radical albeit reconstructive surgery and contradicts a TNT philosophy aiming at organ preservation for all cases of locally advanced rectal cancer. On the other end of the spectrum, PROSPECT might have resulted in overtreatment. A different approach, more common in England and continental Europe, is initial surgery based on MR results followed by chemotherapy based on specimen pathology [2]. Initial surgery would address overtreatment. I feel though that the TNT data indicates a benefit in reducing distant disease, which presumably indicates that preoperative chemotherapy, as part of TNT, is more effective than postoperative chemotherapy. I feel more inclined to give the benefit of the doubt to the favorable effect of upfront chemotherapy and accept the inevitable proportion of overtreated patients. We have already moved from postoperative radiotherapy to preoperative radiotherapy in rectal cancer, and we remain well aware of the associated risk of overtreatment. We can do the same with neoadjuvant chemotherapy.

References

1. Morton D, Seymour M, Magill L, Handley K, Glasbey J, Glimelius B, Palmer A, Seligmann J, Laurberg S, Murakami K, West N, Quirke P, Gray R; FOxTROT Collaborative Group. Preoperative chemotherapy for operable colon cancer: mature results of an international randomized controlled trial. J Clin Oncol. 2023;41(8):1541–1552.
2. Ruppert R, Junginger T, Kube R, Strassburg J, Lewin A, Baral J, Maurer CA, Sauer J, Lauscher J, Winde G, Thomasmeyer R, Stelzner S, Bambauer C, Scheunemann S, Faedrich A, Wollschlaeger D, Merkel S. Risk-adapted neoadjuvant Chemoradiotherapy in rectal cancer: final report of the OCUM study. J Clin Oncol. 2023;41(24):4025–4034.

Discussion

LS

Amit, I remember we had a conversation at one of our Journal club meetings when discussing this article, and I remember you said that PROSPECT is obsolete, which is a valid criticism, I think, but please just speak your mind.

AM

Yes. What I believe about PROSPECT is that it is a great thing that it is a randomized trial which accrued some 1200 odd patients, a giant randomized trial on rectal cancer, which I think is very difficult to achieve, but it also took over 10 years to obtain the data, and in that time frame, other new paradigms of rectal cancer treatment arose. The whole concept of nonoperative management took flight. And so, in general, to me, in the era of watch-and-wait and nonoperative management and obtaining a complete clinical response, that is what potentially makes the PROSPECT trial relatively obsolete. I think it has demonstrated that in selected patients, obviously omitting chemoradiotherapy is appropriate, and I think its applicability is dependent upon our goal for the patient treatment.

LS

Also, the issue that I think pertains to perhaps the Mayo Clinic is that if an individual consults on the Web "Ask the Mayo expert" the recommendation there is that if the patient can be operated on with a restorative procedure, then they would not be a candidate for nonoperative management, and this is exactly the subgroup of patients who were included in this trial, as eligibility criterion; otherwise, they would not enter PROSPECT. Do you feel that this would make the trial more suitable for such a practice, meaning the exclusion from nonoperative management in case of a restorative procedure or are you referring more to the concept of TNT?

AM

My comments are in general more applied to the concept of TNT and how the paradigm has already shifted toward TNT for basically any patient that requires neoadjuvant therapy regardless of whether our goal is to obtain complete response or not. So, I think that's part of it. I think our general Mayo Clinic position on the concept of watch-and-wait has been, I think, more conservative in terms of those that are reconstructible without necessarily pursuing watch-and-wait all the times. Yes, PROSPECT gives us some more data and an opportunity to solidify our basis for treatment recommendations, where historically we have tended to be aggressive in avoiding or trying to avoid radiation therapy, particularly for upper rectal cancers.

MD

I agree that the paradigm has indeed shifted from the conception of this study to its completion and publication, particularly regarding TNT and watch-and-wait strategies. However, I still believe that the data presented are crucial in advocating against the indiscriminate use of radiation therapy in cases of upper and mid-rectal cancers. As surgeons, we often overlook the potential long-term consequences of radiation in these patients. Specifically, for mid-rectal cancers, the inclusion of radiation significantly impacts their long-term functional outcomes. Therefore, these findings serve as valuable support for opting for chemotherapy alone in patients who exhibit a favorable response to such treatment, particularly when watch-and-wait strategies are not pursued.

DC

This is another noninferiority trial with all the caveats that are inherent to it, interpreting the data certainly is something that has been challenging in the past. In essence, this trial shows that if you do have a patient who is absolutely against any radiation, for whatever reason (and I have seen patients with this reluctance to radiation), you have an alternative. Or if they already have issues with continence, and you think radiation will worsen that significantly. In addition, this trial looked at T2N+ disease, T3N− disease, and T3N+ disease, so our discussions and application are limited to these patients.

Total Neoadjuvant Treatment and Organ Preservation in Rectal Cancer

15

Garcia-Aguilar J, Patil S, Gollub MJ, et al. Organ preservation in patients with rectal adenocarcinoma treated with total neoadjuvant therapy. J Clin Oncol. 2022;40(23):2546–2556.

Abstract

Purpose: Prospective data on the efficacy of a watch-and-wait strategy to achieve organ preservation in patients with locally advanced rectal cancer treated with total neoadjuvant therapy are limited.

Methods: In this prospective, randomized phase II trial, we assessed the outcomes of 324 patients with stage II or III rectal adenocarcinoma treated with induction chemotherapy followed by chemoradiotherapy (INCT-CRT) or chemoradiotherapy followed by consolidation chemotherapy (CRT-CNCT) and either total mesorectal excision (TME) or watch-and-wait on the basis of tumor response. Patients in both groups received 4 months of infusional fluorouracil–leucovorin–oxaliplatin or capecitabine–oxaliplatin and 5000–5600 cGy of radiation combined with either continuous infusion fluorouracil or capecitabine during radiotherapy. The trial was designed as two stand-alone studies with disease-free survival (DFS) as the primary endpoint for both groups, with a comparison to a null hypothesis on the basis of historical data. The secondary endpoint was TME-free survival.

© The Author(s), under exclusive license to Springer Nature Switzerland AG 2025
D. Colibaseanu et al., *Essential Articles in Colorectal Surgery*,
https://doi.org/10.1007/978-3-031-77745-5_15

Results: Median follow-up was 3 years. Three-year DFS was 76% (95% CI, 69–84) for the INCT-CRT group and 76% (95% CI, 69–83) for the CRT-CNCT group, in line with the 3-year DFS rate (75%) observed historically. Three-year TME-free survival was 41% (95% CI, 33–50) in the INCT-CRT group and 53% (95% CI, 45–62) in the CRT-CNCT group. No differences were found between groups in local recurrence-free survival, distant metastasis-free survival, or overall survival. Patients who underwent TME after restaging and patients who underwent TME after regrowth had similar DFS rates.

Conclusion: Organ preservation is achievable in half of the patients with rectal cancer treated with total neoadjuvant therapy, without an apparent detriment in survival, compared with historical controls treated with chemoradiotherapy, TME, and postoperative chemotherapy.

LS

This is a trial which has led to widespread change in clinical practice. The investigators treated stage II or III rectal cancers with total neoadjuvant therapy (TNT) and randomized 324 patients to induction chemotherapy-chemoradiotherapy (INCT-CRT) vs. chemoradiotherapy-consolidation chemotherapy (CRT-CNCT). Patients were re-evaluated 8 weeks (±4) following TNT completion. Patients experiencing partial response were recommended to have surgery through total mesorectal excision (TME), while cases with clinical complete response (cCR) were enrolled into a watch-and-wait (WW) protocol. The option of WW was also offered to patients experiencing near-complete clinical response. The initial results at 3 years indicated that in about 50% of patients, it was possible to pursue WW with organ preservation. The updated results are based on a median follow-up of 5.1 years among patients who were alive and event-free at the time of the analysis. The total mesorectal excision (TME)-free survival was 39% in the INCT-CRT group versus 54% in the CRT-CNCT group. The difference in organ preservation favoring CRT-CNCT was also detected in the original trial and is still debated. One of the possible explanations for this difference is that the median time from completion of CRT to restaging was 28.5 weeks in the CRT-CNCT group vs. 8 weeks in the INCT-CRT group. The 5-year disease-free survival rates were similar among INCT-CRT and CRT-CNCT (71% and 69%, respectively). Among the 25% of patients (81/324) experiencing tumor regrowth, 94% of these events occurred within 2 years after completion of TNT. Disease-free survival was 64% in both patients who underwent TME after restaging and patients initially managed with watchful waiting who underwent TME after tumor regrowth [1]. The design of the OPRA trial builds on the pioneering work on WW and organ preservation in rectal cancer by Habr-Gama [2]. As a large, well-designed prospective American trial, OPRA has led to a more definitive recognition of the role of nonoperative management of rectal cancer with organ preservation which is now included in the NCCN guidelines [3]. This greatly facilitates my practice since WW is now one of the accepted treatment approaches at least in case of cCR. I am relieved I no longer must warn patients asking me for this specific approach that despite all its merits, WW is outside the current standards of care. One of the limitations of WW is the intensive follow-up. It included in the OPRA study flexible sigmoidoscopy every 4 months for the first 2 years and every 6 months for the following 3 years and rectal MR every 6 months for the first 2 years and yearly for the following 3 years at a minimum. There were study patients who were even evaluated at more frequent intervals if this was considered necessary. This can be logistically daunting for some patients. In addition, not all patients in the United States might have insurance coverage for so many frequent evaluations. However, the data indicate that the risk of regrowth rate is much higher in the first 2 years after TNT thus requiring frequent monitoring. Despite its increasing acceptance there are still many surgeons who are comfortable in recommending WW after cCR has been achieved but remain concerned about offering WW in case of near-complete response which is associated with a higher rate of tumor regrowth when compared to WW after cCR. On the other hand, organ preservation is an enormously attractive option to patients, especially for those who would otherwise require a permanent colostomy. Some surgeons are still skeptical of WW if the tumor can be treated with a restorative resection, although a small study has indicated that WW was associated with better anorectal functional results when compared to a matched group of patients undergoing sphincter-sparing TME [4]. Future studies will need to focus on optimized combination treatments, including the possible role of short-course radiotherapy, and simplified surveillance approaches. However, in one form or another, I feel that WW is here to stay.

References

1. Verheij FS, Omer DM, Williams H, Lin ST, Qin LX, Buckley JT, Thompson HM, Yuval JB, Kim JK, Dunne RF, Marcet J, Cataldo P, Polite B, Herzig DO, Liska D, Oommen S, Friel CM, Ternent C, Coveler AL, Hunt S, Gregory A, Varma MG, Bello BL, Carmichael JC, Krauss J, Gleisner A, Guillem JG, Temple L, Goodman KA, Segal NH, Cercek A, Yaeger R, Nash GM, Widmar M, Wei IH, Pappou EP, Weiser MR, Paty PB, Smith JJ, Wu AJ, Gollub MJ, Saltz LB, Garcia-Aguilar J. Long-term results of organ preservation in patients with rectal adenocarcinoma treated with Total neoadjuvant therapy: the randomized phase II OPRA trial. J Clin Oncol. 2024;42(5):500–506.
2. Habr-Gama A, Perez RO, Nadalin W, et al. Operative versus nonoperative treatment for stage 0 distal rectal cancer following chemoradiation therapy: long-term results. Ann Surg. 2004;240:711–718.
3. Benson AB, Venook AP, Al-Hawary MM, Azad N, Chen YJ, Ciombor KK, Cohen S, Cooper HS, Deming D, Garrido-Laguna I, Grem JL, Gunn A, Hecht JR, Hoffe S, Hubbard J, Hunt S, Jeck W, Johung KL, Kirilcuk N, Krishnamurthi S, Maratt JK, Messersmith WA, Meyerhardt J, Miller ED, Mulcahy MF, Nurkin S, Overman MJ, Parikh A, Patel H, Pedersen K, Saltz L, Schneider C, Shibata D, Skibber JM, Sofocleous CT, Stotsky-Himelfarb E, Tavakkoli A, Willett CG, Gregory K, Gurski L. Rectal cancer, version 2.2022, NCCN

clinical practice guidelines in oncology. J Natl Compr Canc Netw. 2022;20(10):1139–1167.

4. Quezada-Diaz FF, Smith JJ, Jimenez-Rodriguez RM, Wasserman I, Pappou EP, Patil S, Wei IH, Nash GM, Guillem JG, Weiser MR, Paty PB, Garcia-Aguilar J. Patient-reported bowel function in patients with rectal cancer managed by a watch-and-wait strategy after neoadjuvant therapy: a case-control study. Dis Colon Rectum. 2020;63(7): 897–902.

Discussion

AM

I think organ preservation and nonoperative management are the future of rectal cancer treatment. When comparing this with PROSPECT, it seems like we went through this shift of no radiation to radiation plus chemotherapy, from trying to omit radiation to now bringing everything upfront through every possible treatment combination to achieve complete response and nonoperative management. Obviously, this only reports disease-free survival. But really the key factor is the outcome of those patients who experience regrowth who then undergo TME, and then, is there an impact on their survival? And what is their true change in survival? I think the long-term results of OPRA were just published in February 2024, and the TME-free survival was still high, but greater with consolidation chemotherapy, 54% vs. 39% with induction chemotherapy, and that was statistically significant. The other interesting thing with the long-term results is when are they going to regrow? And how do you then follow these people who have achieved complete clinical response? 90–95% of those with recurrence/regrowth had it within 2 years, and then, like 99% or 100% had occurred within 3 years. And so, I think those that fail, you tend to know pretty early, and overall, they still have very good long-term results with avoiding surgery. Again, to me, it all boils down to patient selection and patient counseling in terms of outcomes in the setting of regrowth and subsequent surgery, and some of that is still unknown.

LS

The long-term results do indicate that survival is similar between patients who are treated with salvage TME following regrowth vs. initial TME after treatment, right?

AM

Disease-free survival, but we do not know overall survival.

LS

Yes.

DC

From a skeptic's perspective, the issue here is that we still have 160 patients or so in each arm, so there is not going to be a lot of patients. So, we have to take these results with a grain of salt. And then, not insignificant is the fact that the surveillance is absolutely necessary and rather intense. Having an MRI every 6 months for the first 2 years is something that patients have to sign up for. So, this is not necessarily for everybody. It would be something for a motivated patient who can continue intense surveillance tests and follow-up visits. So, I am happy that this trial was done, and I am excited about the promise that it brings, but I just think that we need to take it with a grain of salt and take it for what it is with the shortcomings that the treatment potentially has.

MD

I think that the results of this trial are very exciting with regard to the nonoperative management of rectal cancer. What was interesting in this trial was the number of patients who were offered watch-and-wait, which was about 75% in both arms, which I think is an extraordinarily high number, although they did include patients with near-complete response. I think it would be interesting to differentiate how those with near complete vs. complete response did, and I did not get that from the study. The study also indicated that consolidation chemotherapy is a better choice when we are trying to achieve a complete response as opposed to induction chemotherapy, which is an important conversation to have with patients prior to treatment initiation. For you folks, how comfortable do you feel offering watch-and-wait to patients with near complete response? And how do you define endoscopically what a near complete response is?

AM

To me, all of it is largely driven by the patient in most situations. When it is near complete versus even in the setting of complete response. All of this is driven by the patient so much, but at least less so by us, I think, as providers, because I think we have a natural bias in favor of surgery. Most of us do, I think. And when I say us, I mean the colorectal community at large is only now starting to shift, I think, toward some more widespread acceptance of watch-and-wait. For your second question, I think what constitutes near complete response has yet to be really defined appropriately. I mean, we are only now better understanding and seeing published information on the standardization of the definition of complete response. Flat white scar telangiectasia vs. maybe a near complete response. I just read about near complete response described as a single, solitary ulceration. I think that part of the problem is that we have not defined standards in the description of near-complete response. And also, I am thinking, what are the standards of evaluation in the setting of near complete response, how do you follow these patients? At what interval should you get imaging, or should you not? It has already been accepted that you should not really biopsy lesions because of the risk of sampling error. And do you believe a negative biopsy? I think that is an area where there is still a lot to be known or learned.

LS

I would say nodules and ulcer for example, if the lining of the mucosa has any bumps, that to me excludes the idea of complete clinical response. As far as my comfort level in continuing watch-and-wait, not as comfortable but because there are data I mention this to patients and to echo Amit's comments, the patient largely drives this, so I just write in my note something to the effect that this is still an uncharted territory. Now, we have clinical guidelines on clinical complete response. We do not have clinical guidelines on near-complete response. We have data, especially from Memorial Sloan Kettering, indicating that near-complete response could progress to complete response over time. I have continued watching patients with near-complete response at three-month intervals. That has been my practice so far, and hopefully, in the future, we will have more definitive data as we have now on clinical complete response. I avoid biopsies in this setting for the reasons you outlined.

DC

Another comment about this, not on the study itself, but on the consequences of continuing this trend of watch-and-wait. There is some import to the trainees. We already have some training centers that do less rectal cancer surgeries than I think should-to sufficiently train the colorectal surgery fellows. This will make rectal cancer surgery scarcer, and outside of tertiary centers, it will be hard to train fellows. Not that we should avoid implementing a better treatment because we need to train surgeons, but it is something we will have to contend with within the next 5 years, or earlier.

AM

I think what will be interesting to look at is also rates of sphincter preservation. I mean, we see it in these papers specifically looking at watch-and-wait, but we published an NCDB study looking at rates of sphincter preservation. It was very similar to the rates reported in Rocco Ricciardi's earlier papers examining a variety of other databases, and it has always hovered between 23 and 25% abdomino-perineal resection rate for rectal cancers across all stages. So, it will be interesting to revisit the NCDB (National Cancer DataBase) data on the abdomino-perineal resection rate as the watch-and-wait practice becomes more mature to see if that will change. I think the paper we wrote was from 2017.

LS

I agree. As we said though, this trend is also largely patient-driven. I mean, you have patients that come in, and they might not be necessarily very sophisticated, but they already know about this, and they ask if we can treat their disease without giving them a bag. So, I think that there is a lot of pressure to apply watch-and-wait, which will also help in understanding its limitations and establishing it as a viable practice.

Short-Course Vs. Long-Course Radiotherapy Before Chemotherapy and Surgery for Rectal Cancer

16

Dijkstra EA, Nilsson PJ, Hospers GAP, Bahadoer RR, Meershoek-Klein Kranenbarg E, Roodvoets AGH, Putter H, Berglund Å, Cervantes A, Crolla RMPH, Hendriks MP, Capdevila J, Edhemovic I, Marijnen CAM, van de Velde CJH, Glimelius B, van Etten B; Collaborative Investigators. Locoregional failure during and after short-course radiotherapy followed by chemotherapy and surgery compared with long-course chemoradiotherapy and surgery: a 5-year follow-up of the RAPIDO trial. Ann Surg. 2023;278(4):e766–e772.

Abstract

Objective: To analyze risk and patterns of locoregional failure (LRF) in patients of the RAPIDO trial at 5 years.

Background: Multimodality treatment improves local control in rectal cancer. Total neoadjuvant treatment (TNT) aims to improve systemic control while local control is maintained. At 3 years, LRF rate was comparable between TNT and chemoradiotherapy in the RAPIDO trial.

Methods: A total of 920 patients were randomized between an experimental (EXP, short-course radiotherapy, chemotherapy, and surgery) and a standard-care group (STD, chemoradiotherapy, surgery, and optional postoperative chemotherapy). LRFs, including early LRF (no resection except for organ preservation/R2

© The Author(s), under exclusive license to Springer Nature Switzerland AG 2025
D. Colibaseanu et al., *Essential Articles in Colorectal Surgery*, https://doi.org/10.1007/978-3-031-77745-5_16

resection) and locoregional recurrence (LRR) after an R0/R1 resection, were analyzed.

Results: Totally, 460 EXP and 446 STD patients were eligible. At 5.6 years (median follow-up), LRF was detected in 54/460 (12%) and 36/446 (8%) patients in the EXP and STD groups, respectively ($P = 0.07$), in which EXP patients were more often treated with three-dimensional-conformed radiotherapy ($P = 0.029$). In the EXP group, LRR was detected more often [44/431 (10%) vs. 26/428 (6%); $P = 0.027$], with more often a breached mesorectum (9/44 (21%) vs. 1/26 (4); $P = 0.048$). The EXP treatment, enlarged lateral lymph nodes, positive circumferential resection margin, tumor deposits, and node positivity at pathology were the significant predictors for developing LRR. Location of the LRRs was similar between groups. Overall survival after LRF was comparable [hazard ratio: 0.76 (95% CI, 0.46–1.26); $P = 0.29$].

Conclusions: The EXP treatment was associated with an increased risk of LRR, whereas the reduction in disease-related treatment failure and distant metastases remained after 5 years. Further refinement of the TNT in rectal cancer is mandated.

LS

This could be viewed as a large trial which assessed total neoadjuvant treatment (TNT) using short-course radiotherapy. The experimental arm consisted of short-course radiotherapy and chemotherapy before radical surgery, while the comparative standard arm consisted of long-course chemoradiotherapy, surgery, and optional postoperative chemotherapy. The trial was successful in that its results at 5 years confirm the previously reported significant association between experimental treatment and reduction in both disease-related treatment failure and distant metastasis rates. However, the trial has been criticized in its design with respect to the radiotherapy technique, the interval between TNT and surgery, and because its endpoints were changed over time. In particular, disease-free survival was abandoned as an outcome of interest in favor of disease-related treatment failure [1]. In addition, overall survival was similar, although this is not necessarily surprising as some oncologic outcomes require longer follow-ups to result in statistically different mortality rates. From a more strictly surgical perspective, local recurrence was significantly more common in the short-course radiotherapy plus chemotherapy group, although the difference barely achieved statistical significance. Importantly, the cases of local recurrences in the experimental arm were also more commonly associated with a mesorectal breach, which has raised concerns on the deleterious effect on the operative field deriving from a longer interval between short-course radiotherapy and surgery [2]. Given these results, surgeons accustomed to long-course chemoradiotherapy may feel uncomfortable at the idea of just switching to short-course radiotherapy for the same indications. This is particularly the case for high-risk locally advanced rectal cancer patients such as some of those accrued into RAPIDO. The integration of long-course chemoradiotherapy, total neoadjuvant treatment, and possible nonoperative management is now part of accepted guidelines, and we also have important information on regrowth risk and regrowth rate over time as well as expected results of salvage surgery. If we assume that long-course and short-course radiotherapy are *per se* equivalent, it would seem logical that surgeons who are more familiar with short-course radiotherapy would be more interested in a total neoadjuvant therapy approach retaining their radiotherapy modality of choice. With all its limitations, RAPIDO remains at least a confirmatory trial on the suitability and effectiveness of total neoadjuvant treatment which was associated with a 28% pathologic complete response rate [3]. At the time of its implementation, the experience with watch-and-wait was limited in Europe, and therefore, this was not included as an option already embedded into the trial design [4]. The experience accumulated in RAPIDO can now inform the design of future trials also examining nonoperative management.

References

1. Riou O, Gourgou S, Conroy T. Comment on "Locoregional failure during and after short-course radiotherapy followed by chemotherapy and surgery compared to long-course chemoradiotherapy and surgery: a five-year follow-up of the RAPIDO trial": the RAPIDO trial does not achieve its primary endpoint. Ann Surg Open. 2023;4(2):e288.
2. Glynne-Jones R, Hollingshead J. TNT and local recurrence in the RAPIDO trial—untangling the puzzle. Nat Rev Clin Oncol. 2023;20(6):357–358.
3. Bahadoer RR, Dijkstra EA, van Etten B, Marijnen CAM, Putter H, Kranenbarg EM, Roodvoets AGH, Nagtegaal ID, Beets-Tan RGH, Blomqvist LK, Fokstuen T, Ten Tije AJ, Capdevila J, Hendriks MP, Edhemovic I, Cervantes A, Nilsson PJ, Glimelius B, van de Velde CJH, Hospers GAP; RAPIDO Collaborative Investigators. Short-course radiotherapy followed by chemotherapy before total mesorectal excision (TME) versus preoperative chemoradiotherapy, TME, and optional adjuvant chemotherapy in locally advanced rectal cancer (RAPIDO): a randomised, open-label, phase 3 trial. Lancet Oncol. 2021;22(1):29–42.
4. Nilsson PJ, van Etten B, Hospers GAP, Marijnen CAM, Meershoek-Klein Kranenberg E, Roodvoets AGH, van de Velde CJH, Glimelius B. Comment on the RAPIDO trial point-counterpoint debate. Dis Colon Rectum. 2024;67(2):e126.

Discussion

AM

I think the early results of RAPIDO from the original paper were encouraging, but their conclusions I thought were rather bold in that this whole paradigm and the experimental treatment could be considered as a new standard, as they called it. I thought that was rather bold and premature, which I think was confirmed by the follow-up paper which showed that loco-regional recurrence was worse than in the control group which was statistically significant. And the biggest thing probably related, in my opinion, to the timing of surgery after short-course radiotherapy was an incomplete mesorectum or poor quality surgery at a far higher rate; I think it was 21% compared to 4%. I think TNT is the new standard paradigm for the treatment of rectal cancer but probably not in the order that is described by the RAPIDO trial.

MD

As you said, it was a little bit more promising with their initial results, and certainly with their 5-year follow-up, I would not use short course and specifically in the tumors that they studied, which were more locally advanced T4 tumors or patients with disease in the lateral lymph node compartments. And, in the era of TNT, this study really compared short course and TNT vs. long course and adjuvant chemotherapy, which is not really what the most common practice is now in the era of watch-and-wait and TNT. I think a study looking at short course and TNT compared with long course and TNT would be a little more helpful given how our practices run now.

DC

I think that changing the independent variable (outcome) from one study to the next made me uncomfortable. I think I understand the reason, but mitigating confounders is hard enough even in prospective studies, and this brings in more uncertainty. This certainly has not convinced me to use more short-course radiotherapy, though I admit there are circumstances where it is better to use short course. I thought after reading the original study and before reading the follow-up study that this would sway me in favor of short course, but it did not.

LS

I agree with you. I think it's difficult for anybody but at least for me to shift to some treatment modality which I'm not so accustomed to, and use it regularly to begin with. This is the case for me and short-course radiation treatment. It is an option, and we use it selectively, but it's not our preferred option for most cases of locally advanced rectal cancer, and clearly, this group of investigators explore in their trial the option that they're more comfortable and accustomed to. This is in part the same group that produced, 20 years ago, the Dutch trial. And they are not really the same investigators, but they're basically coming from the same school of thought. And I think that when approaching TNT, they think in terms of TNT with the radiation piece that they are accustomed to, and so their modus operandi is not the result of an abstract choice between long course vs. short course, but it's related to what they're accustomed to. As important as it is, this trial feels a little obsolete in that it was not designed with the TNT and watch-and-wait parts, which I think is how new trials should be designed. And perhaps you could do TNT using short-course radiotherapy and have similar watch-and-weight results as if you do the long-course radiotherapy. So this trial sort of confirms my bias against short course in this patient population. Maybe if short course had been given in a different sequence before surgery, it could have been different. The positive part of the trial is that it confirms the value of TNT for the patient, but for the surgeon, it is concerning for the reasons that Amit outlined.

AM

I think the issues that lead to the negative aspects of RAPIDO revolve on the timing of surgery after the short-course radiotherapy because it was after a prolonged interval. They had radiotherapy, followed by six cycles of CAPOX and then ultimately surgery. So, even beyond 6 weeks. And so it was that prolonged period of time between radiation and surgery where,

I think, anecdotally we say, the rectal dissection is more difficult after short course than long course. I think short course has a role, it definitely has a role, and practices for a long time out of Europe have included it. I think the historic reasons we haven't adopted it in the United States have largely been based on reimbursement because you get paid per fractionation in the United States. And so that's why there was this big push, everything has to be long course, chemoradiotherapy, etc. but I think the role for short course is in patients who don't need significant downstaging in whom there isn't the risk of positive circumferential margin, or when decreasing the size of the tumor is not necessarily going to help significantly with surgery, but maybe it's just sterilizing the pelvis for you. Those are, to me, indications for short course. Still providing the therapy, but then with early surgery, as opposed to the prolonged waiting period, and I think it's in those situations you probably would not see the same issues with mesorectal preservation.

The Role of Diverting Loop Ileostomy as an Adjunct to Low Anterior Resection for Rectal Cancer

17

Matthiessen P, Hallböök O, Rutegård J, Simert G, Sjödahl R. Defunctioning stoma reduces symptomatic anastomotic leakage after low anterior resection of the rectum for cancer: a randomized multicenter trial. Ann Surg. 2007;246(2):207–14.

Abstract

Objective: The aim of this randomized multicenter trial was to assess the rate of symptomatic anastomotic leakage in patients operated on with low anterior resection for rectal cancer and who were intraoperatively randomized to a defunctioning stoma or not.

Summary of Background Data: The introduction of total mesorectal excision surgery as the surgical technique of choice for carcinoma in the lower and mid rectum has led to decreased local recurrence and improved oncological results. Despite these advances, perioperative morbidity remains a major issue, and the most feared complication is symptomatic anastomotic leakage. The role of the defunctioning stoma in regard to anastomotic leakage is controversial and has not been assessed in any randomized trial of sufficient size.

Methods: From December 1999 to June 2005, a total of 234 patients were randomized to a defunctioning loop stoma or no loop stoma. Loop ileostomy or loop transverse colostomy was at the choice of the surgeon. Inclusion criteria for randomization

© The Author(s), under exclusive license to Springer Nature Switzerland AG 2025

D. Colibaseanu et al., *Essential Articles in Colorectal Surgery*,
https://doi.org/10.1007/978-3-031-77745-5_17

were expected survival 6 months, informed consent, anastomosis 7 cm above the anal verge, negative air leakage test, intact anastomotic rings, and absence of major intraoperative adverse events.

Results: The overall rate of symptomatic leakage was 19.2% (45 of 234). Patients randomized to a defunctioning stoma (n = 116) had leakage in 10.3% (12 of 116) and those without stoma (n = 118) in 28.0% (33 of 118) (odds ratio 3.4; 95% confidence interval, 1.6–6.9; $P < 0.001$). The need for urgent abdominal reoperation was 8.6% (10 of 116) in those randomized to stoma and 25.4% (30 of 118) in those without ($P < 0.001$). After a follow-up of median 42 months (range, 6–72 months), 13.8% (16 of 116) of the initially defunctioned patients still had a stoma of any kind, compared with 16.9% (20 of 118) those not defunctioned (not significant). The 30-day mortality after anterior resection was 0.4% (1 of 234) and after elective reversal of a defunctioning stoma was 0.9% (1 of 111). Median age was 68 years (range, 32–86 years), 45.3% (106 of 234) were females, 79.1% (185 of 234) had preoperative radiotherapy, the level of anastomosis was median 5 cm, and intraoperative blood loss 550 mL, without differences between the groups.

Conclusion: Defunctioning loop stoma decreased the rate of symptomatic anastomotic leakage and is therefore recommended in low anterior resection for rectal cancer.

LS

During surgical training, I was taught that the benefit of diverting loop ileostomy after low anterior resection consisted in the reduction in the severity of postoperative infection should an anastomotic leak occur. In addition, it was pointed out to us that a diverting loop ileostomy was not associated with a reduction in the risk of anastomotic leak itself. This was not just some surgeon's personal opinion, and there is evidence supporting this contention [1]. This is the first article that I know of which actually questioned that very tenet with the authority coming from a prospective randomized trial. The authors accrued 234 patients undergoing low anterior resection for rectal adenocarcinoma who were assigned to defunctioning stoma versus no stoma diversion. Patients having a defunctioning stoma were associated with a significantly decreased clinical anastomotic leak rate when compared to those without a stoma (10.3% vs. 28%). The need for urgent abdominal reoperation was correspondingly decreased in the stoma diversion group. There were 2 deaths, 1 after anterior resection and 1 after the takedown of a defunctioning stoma. After a median follow-up of 42 months, the proportion of patients still having a stoma of any kind was similar between groups. The argument could be made that the anastomotic leak rate among patients without a stoma creation was relatively high, thus contributing to the detected statistically significant difference when compared with the defunctionalized group. Perhaps, with a clinical anastomotic leak rate of less than 28%, the difference between groups might have been statistically similar. However, there is more ample evidence suggesting that a diverting stoma is associated with reduced anastomotic leak rate. In a meta-analysis by Emile and coll. based on 9 randomized trials on low anterior resection including 946 patients, the diverting stoma group was associated with a significantly decreased risk of anastomotic leak, whose crude rates could be calculated through the study tables as 7.8% vs. 18.8%, as well as abscess, overall complications, and reoperation rates when compared to low anterior resection without diversion. In addition, the study identified factors significantly associated with an anastomotic leak in non-diverted patients which included increased body mass index, American Society of Anesthesiologists score of 3 or above, more distal location of rectal tumors, use of neoadjuvant therapy, open surgery, end-to-end anastomosis, and longer operative times [2]. None of these factors should be surprising to the practicing surgeon. The other issue related to diversion which points out the consequences of the severity rather than the occurrence of an anastomotic leak *per se* is the case of a patient having a low anastomosis without diversion who might require a takedown of the entire anastomosis due to anastomotic leak, leaving a very short anorectal stump. This is a situation where a future re-establishment of intestinal continuity becomes gravely imperiled, arguably because the surgeon decided against elective stoma diversion at the time of index surgery. It is possible that an anastomotic leak in a diverted patient never heals to the point of allowing takedown of the diverting stoma, which was the case in 13.8% among the initially defunctionalized patients in the prospective randomized trial here presented. However, the chances that the anastomotic leak progressively heals without taking down the entire anastomosis are higher. Therefore, and as pointed out in the commentary to another article, it is prudent to add a stoma diversion to any low anastomosis created during low anterior resection.

References

1. Wong NY, Eu KW. A defunctioning ileostomy does not prevent clinical anastomotic leak after a low anterior resection: a prospective, comparative study. Dis Colon Rectum. 2005;48(11):2076–9.
2. Emile SH, Khan SM, Garoufalia Z, Silva-Alvarenga E, Gefen R, Horesh N, Freund MR, Wexner SD. When is a diverting stoma indicated after low anterior resection? A meta-analysis of randomized trials and meta-regression of the risk factors of leakage and complications in non-diverted patients. J Gastrointest Surg. 2022;26(11):2368–2379.

Discussion

DC

Though a small study, this is an important study, nonetheless. Their selection criteria were interesting, especially the randomization. Out of the 65 hospitals that were included in the study, only 234 patients were randomized over a 5.5-year period. This seems low until you see that over 70% of the patients that were eligible for randomization were not actually randomized for various reasons, but ¼ of them had to have a stoma and thus were not eligible for the study.

This is interesting, because even in the cases in which the surgeons think that a stoma might not be necessary (i.e., preselected cases), almost 20% have leaks. And of those, ¼ of the leaks without a diversion stoma had to have urgent surgery vs. less than 10% in the defunctionalized group.

So as a group, or a systematic approach, the scales are tilted toward a defunctionalizing stoma in LARs, I think. Obviously, there are caveats upon caveats, but this seems the safest general approach if one were to approach the question wholesale.

MD

I think that the study certainly showed that with regard to symptomatic leak, having a defunctionalized stoma decreases that rate. I don't think it really answered the question about asymptomatic leaks because they didn't look at all anastomoses during the time period prior to ileostomy closure to see if there were any occult asymptomatic leaks that perhaps resolved by the time they closed the ileostomy. I thought what was interesting was that they randomized patients to stoma vs. no stoma based essentially on the level of anastomosis of less than 7 cm from the anal verge, but they didn't take into account radiotherapy, something for which I think routinely, at least in my practice, and I know in many people's practices we create a diverting stoma. This could have contributed to the higher leak rate seen in the paper. The authors did mention that they did look at the impact of radiation therapy versus no radiation and didn't see a difference in the anastomotic leak rate. That was the one aspect of the paper that I thought was a little bit different from what standard practice currently is with regard to diversion.

AM

When we're all in training we're, I think, taught a set of rules on when to divert, when not to divert. At least, to me, it seemed like those were a set of rules that were taught as a dictum and not necessarily as a line that is sometimes blurred. I think the decision of diversion versus not diversion is less some set numbers in terms of the height of an anastomosis or radiation vs. no radiation, but more of an overall gestalt of what's going on. So, for example, I don't think it's necessarily mandatory to divert all patients in the setting of past radiation therapy, and this is a personal belief, or for all patients with immunosuppression or for all anastomoses below the anterior perineal reflection. I think you have to take a number of factors into account and make an overall judgment call. And in some cases, that judgment call will be correct, and in others, it may not be. In terms of this paper, more specifically, I think it is an awfully high leak rate, as Dorin pointed out, a 20% rate, and so I think that raises my eyebrows a little bit in terms of interpreting some of the data, but it is there to be interpreted, I suppose.

LS

I understand that in theory, in abstract, there can be a debate on whether stoma diversion helps in reducing the virulence of a clinical leak vs. directly reducing the risk of anastomotic leak occurring at all in the first place. Especially in a very low colorectal or colo-anal anastomosis, the virulence of such infection can threaten the preservation of the anastomosis itself and the ability to ultimately reestablish intestinal continuity. In actual practice, I find the abstract diatribe on virulence vs. occurrence of an anastomotic leak not being so critical for actual decision-making.

AM

I think the other part of this decision process of diverting or not diverting is salvage in those that have not been diverted. And there are groups that have written about intentionally not diverting low rectal cancer and at the earliest sign of a leak whether it's obvious or not, then they go and divert them and have a reasonable rate of salvage. Not necessarily something that I do.

LS

This is something that was also proposed after ileal pouch-anal anastomosis. Perhaps because I've never done it, I'm suspicious of this practice. I feel there are a number of situations where the leak is initially subtle in its clinical presentations and by the time it becomes clinically manifest, its virulence is much greater. The other concern I would have is how attentive the monitoring of patients would be especially if the patient deteriorates during night shifts and weekends and how expeditious would the treatment be under those circumstances. This practice would predispose by design to a greater number of such events than routine stoma diversion. Again, I must admit, I have never done this and have not been trained in this, so I ultimately have no experience.

MD

So, in those studies, are they routinely doing radiographic imaging to look at the anastomosis? Or just following clinically after surgery?

AM

I guess both approaches have been described. Like the French group has written about this, where they've just followed them clinically, but patients have a longer length of stay in the hospital, a longer period of time of following them. In those situations, others have used more objective metrics, whether CRP or early imaging. And then there have been kind of the other ancillary group of patients, those undergoing early stoma closure. There have been a few studies indicating that early ileostomy closure is associated with a negative outcome. And those are patients who presumably did not have a clinically identifiable leak at the time. And so, if you think of that patient population now just being devil's advocate about lack of ileostomy creation, those are patients who didn't have a sign of a clinical leak, had an early reversal, and then developed a problem. Makes you question, I guess, the decision of leaving a low anastomosis undiverted.

MD

So, what do you guys do in your practice? Based on some of the data we have, I generally will divert those patients who have low anastomoses less than seven centimeters from the anal verge and underwent radiotherapy. Either or, not necessarily both. I like applying both criteria. In what instance are you guys not diverting? Radiated or low anastomosis?

AM

For me, it is not necessarily a number in terms of height, but where the anastomosis is in relation to the anterior peritoneal reflection. If the anastomosis is below the peritoneal reflection, there is a far higher likelihood, I'm diverting them versus if it's above. And, I don't know, just maybe it's my own psychosis about it. I just draw it as a line in the sand if it's above, and if it's only a centimeter above, it's still above to me. If it's 5 cm above, it's above. If it's a centimeter below, it is below. For me, that's probably the biggest determining factor. And then second, I would guess, the delivery of radiation. But, for example, the transplant patient population in which we operate on frequently, and this may not necessarily be related to cancer and directly relevant to this paper, is a population that's on immunosuppressives. To me, those patients don't necessarily mandate a diversion just because they're on immunosuppression. Again, probably the biggest factor for me is relation to the anterior peritoneal reflection.

DC

Yeah, I'd say for me—at least conceptually—it's not necessarily a specific anatomical set point. It is an evaluation of how much tension there is on the anastomosis, and what are the consequences of a leak? Can the patient even survive a potential leak, and is the anastomosis so low that the leak jeopardizes any chance of being able to establish intestinal continuity in the future? What is this patient's continence to begin with? I think that the exact distance of the anastomosis from the anal verge is more of a "place holder" or equivalency estimation for these considerations rather than an end onto itself.

LS

I see your points, but I would say, having experienced both the complications of a diverted ileostomy and its closure vs. low anastomosis without proximal diversion, whenever there are any of those factors that you mentioned, I tend to be liberal in diverting because I feel the morbidity associated with a diverting ileostomy and its closure is in general the lesser of the two evils. If somebody is healthy, if their anastomosis is high, without tension, and with a good blood supply, then I do not divert. But in all those circumstances, malnutrition, or if I feel the patient is marginal due to comorbidities, I divert. I have also diverted all patients on immunosuppression for transplant. I recognize that perhaps we should be more selective in the transplant patients and depending on the kind of transplant. Kidney transplant recipients tend to be more similar to the general population than, let's say, lung transplant recipients. So, in a patient with lung transplant, I'm much more concerned about what happens if the patient has postoperative sepsis, so I would tend to be more liberal in creating a stoma diversion.

AM

I think the overall theme is we are all taking into account the entire overall gestalt of what's going on and multiple factors decide. And I also think as you just alluded to, we need to be weighing the risk of diversion vs. the risk of leak although in the acute period; the risk of leak is probably more impactful. However, there is not an insignificant risk related to diversion in some populations.

Laparoscopic vs. Open Proctectomy for Rectal Cancer

18

Fleshman J, Branda M, Sargent DJ, Boller AM, George V, Abbas M, Peters WR Jr., Maun D, Chang G, Herline A, Fichera A, Mutch M, Wexner S, Whiteford M, Marks J, Birnbaum E, Margolin D, Larson D, Marcello P, Posner M, Read T, Monson J, Wren SM, Pisters PW, Nelson H. Effect of laparoscopic-assisted resection vs open resection of stage II or III rectal cancer on pathologic outcomes: the ACOSOG Z6051 randomized clinical trial. JAMA. 2015;314(13):1346–55.

Abstract

Importance: Evidence about the efficacy of laparoscopic resection of rectal cancer is incomplete, particularly for patients with more advanced-stage disease.

Objective: To determine whether laparoscopic resection is noninferior to open resection, as determined by gross pathologic and histologic evaluation of the resected proctectomy specimen.

Design, Setting, and Participants: A multicenter, balanced, noninferiority, randomized trial enrolled patients between October 2008 and September 2013. The trial was conducted by credentialed surgeons from 35 institutions in the United States and Canada. A total of 486 patients with clinical stage II or III rectal cancer within 12 cm of the anal verge were randomized after completion of neoadjuvant therapy to laparoscopic or open resection.

© The Author(s), under exclusive license to Springer Nature Switzerland AG 2025
D. Colibaseanu et al., *Essential Articles in Colorectal Surgery*,
https://doi.org/10.1007/978-3-031-77745-5_18

Interventions: Standard laparoscopic and open approaches were performed by the credentialed surgeons.

Main Outcomes and Measures: The primary outcome assessing efficacy was a composite of circumferential radial margin greater than 1 mm, distal margin without tumor, and completeness of total mesorectal excision. A 6% noninferiority margin was chosen according to clinical relevance estimation.

Results: Two hundred forty patients with laparoscopic resection and 222 with open resection were evaluable for analysis of the 486 enrolled. Successful resection occurred in 81.7% of laparoscopic resection cases (95% CI, 76.8–86.6%) and 86.9% of open resection cases (95% CI, 82.5–91.4%) and did not support noninferiority (difference, −5.3%; 1-sided 95% CI, −10.8% to ∞; P for noninferiority = 0.41). Patients underwent low anterior resection (76.7%) or abdominoperineal resection (23.3%). Conversion to open resection occurred in 11.3% of patients. Operative time was significantly longer for laparoscopic resection (mean, 266.2 vs. 220.6 min; mean difference, 45.5 min; 95% CI, 27.7–63.4; $P < 0.001$). Length of stay (7.3 vs. 7.0 days; mean difference, 0.3 days; 95% CI, −0.6 to 1.1), readmission within 30 days (3.3% vs. 4.1%; difference, −0.7%; 95% CI, −4.2% to 2.7%), and severe complications (22.5% vs. 22.1%; difference, 0.4%; 95% CI, −4.2% to 2.7%) did not differ significantly. Quality of the total mesorectal excision specimen in 462 operated and analyzed surgeries was complete (77%) and nearly complete (16.5%) in 93.5% of the cases. Negative circumferential radial margin was observed in 90% of the overall group (87.9% laparoscopic resection and 92.3% open resection; $P = 0.11$). Distal margin result was negative in more than 98% of patients irrespective of type of surgery ($P = 0.91$).

Conclusions and Relevance: Among patients with stage II or III rectal cancer, the use of laparoscopic resection compared with open resection failed to meet the criterion for noninferiority for pathologic outcomes. Pending clinical oncologic outcomes, the findings do not support the use of laparoscopic resection in these patients.

DC

This was a prospective randomized trial that enrolled patients between October 2008 and September 2013. It was published in JAMA in October 2015.

This was a noninferiority randomized trial involving 35 institutions in N. America (US and Canada). The primary outcome measured was " … efficacy [of obtaining] a composite of circumferential margin greater than 1mm, distal margin without tumor, and completeness of total mesorectal excision (TME)." All three components had to be completed for the surgery to be considered a success.

The patient population was stage II and III rectal cancer patients (at or below 12 cm from the anal verge). Patients could have chemoradiotherapy or radiotherapy alone. The surgery was done 4–12 weeks after completion of radiotherapy by credentialed surgeons who were tested for competency prior to being able to enroll in the study. Ultimately, after randomizing 486 patients, 240 patients finished in the laparoscopic group and 222 in the open surgery. The primary analysis was a modified intent-to-treat; meaning if a patient was randomized to a laparoscopic group but had an open surgery, they remained in the laparoscopic group (27 of the patients in the laparoscopic arm were converted).

The Statistical Analysis

- The basic assumption was that there would be a 90% success in obtaining the primary outcome. So, to obtain an 80% power the sample size needed to be 480 in total, or 240 per arm.

Measuring the Primary Outcome (3 Criteria)

LAR was done in 76.7% of the patients, and APR in 23.3%, respectively. Conversion to an open procedure was seen in 11% of the laparoscopic procedures, and conversion to an APR was seen in

2.7% of cases. No changes in the open cases. The open cases were just over 3.5 h in duration and over 4 h in the laparoscopic group.

Only 77.1% of TME was complete and 16.5% near complete. The negative circumferential margin and negative distal margin were 90% and 98% overall, respectively, with no statistical difference between the groups. However, when taking all three criteria together, "surgical success" was 86.9% in the open resection arm vs. 81.7% in the laparoscopic arm. This net 5.2% noninferiority margin was the source of many discussions and publications subsequently. All that could be said though was that based on this study, the authors could not allege that laparoscopic proctectomies are not inferior based on the 3-requirement outcome surgical criteria.

This study was mirrored by another, similar-sized Australasian study published in the same exact same issue of JAMA [1]. The studies were designed to be similar. These two studies were subsequently used as an example in a subsequent JAMA publication illustrating just how confusing it is to interpret noninferiority studies [2]. The authors state clearly that all a noninferiority trial can tell you is that an intervention is not worse than a comparator. The results of this slightly underpowered study simply could not say that laparoscopic proctectomy is noninferior. The problem here was that in essence, the study was inconclusive. That is the best way to word the results. After all of this work, it is just not clear that there is a difference. Or, if there was a difference, this study does not have sufficient power to pick it up. So, because of that, less than one-quarter of the publications that reference this study accurately and clearly state that the results are inconclusive (of the 130 or so studies that mention either of the two noninferiority studies above). More than one quarter of publications incorrectly interpret the results of these studies, and more than half are somewhat unclear of what their conclusions regarding this study actually are.

What actually happened in practice? Mostly, nothing changed. Some institutions changed their practice, some incorrectly understanding the results of ACOSOC Z6051, and some not being able to justify an additional hour of surgery without clarity on whether laparoscopy is the same or inferior to open surgery. In the end though, the 2-year disease-free interval of the patients enrolled in ACOSOC

Z6051 was published, and there was no difference [3]. Take-home lessons: (1) Non-inferiority studies seem to be a mystery within a question for some when the result is different than the one you expect. (2) To ambiguous results do not clarify the question.

References

1. Stevenson AR, Solomon MJ, Lumley JW, et al.; ALaCaRT Investigators. Effect of laparoscopic-assisted resection vs open resection on pathological outcomes in rectal cancer: the ALaCaRT randomized clinical trial. JAMA. 2015;314(13):1356–1363.
2. Acuna SA, Dossa F, Baxter NN. Frequency of misinterpretation of inconclusive noninferiority trials: the case of the laparoscopic vs open resection for rectal cancer trials. JAMA Surg. 2019;154(1):90–92.
3. Fleshman J, Branda ME, Sargent DJ, Boller AM, George VV, Abbas MA, Peters WR Jr., Maun DC, Chang GJ, Herline A, Fichera A, Mutch MG, Wexner SD, Whiteford MH, Marks J, Birnbaum E, Margolin DA, Larson DW, Marcello PW, Posner MC, Read TE, Monson JRT, Wren SM, Pisters PWT, Nelson H. Disease-free survival and local recurrence for laparoscopic resection compared with open resection of stage II to III rectal cancer: follow-up results of the ACOSOG Z6051 randomized controlled trial. Ann Surg. 2019;269(4):589–595.

Discussion

LS

I find this study very important both in terms of driving clinical practice and also in reaffirming the role of scientific studies in surgery. This was supposed to become the consecration of laparoscopic surgery for rectal cancer on the wave of multiple randomized trials which had established the advantages of laparoscopic surgery for colon cancer. However, the results of this trial were inconclusive in establishing the noninferiority of laparoscopic surgery. Importantly and as you mentioned in your comments, the results of this trial were basically mirrored by the Australasian trial which had a similar design. The combination of these studies could be viewed as a scientific experiment which could be replicated in another laboratory, and this really thwarted my enthusiasm for laparoscopic surgery in rectal cancer. One aspect that was very critical for me as a surgeon was to see that even the recovery benefits traditionally associated with laparoscopic surgery were absent in this trial where the hospital length of stay was statistically similar between the 2 study arms. The honest conclusion at least for the type of patients who had been randomized was that there was simply no good reason to do laparoscopic surgery, which was hard to accept for me as somebody who had actually entered patients into this trial. The oncologic concerns which emerged when the trial was published have not been substantiated by subsequent follow-up studies indicating that there was no difference between laparoscopic and open proctectomy in oncologic outcomes. In retrospect, it is possible that the creation of a composite pathologic outcome including free resection margin and complete or near complete mesorectum was not the ideal surrogate endpoint to be used for this study. With the advent of robotic surgery, this study might seem obsolete, but it remains a cautionary tale on the primacy of science over our own expert opinions and the importance of being humble.

DC

The primary issue is that most people do not know what to do with a noninferiority trial. So, even if the study were perfect with perfect results, some people still would have trouble figuring out what the results mean. Ultimately what one could say for sure is that we cannot say that laparoscopic surgery is in some way better. Some said that, "well, we will just go back to hand-assisted"— which I do not do—and others said that they will just talk to the patient and tell them that we don't know if laparoscopic is better, but we don't even know if it's not worse and we'll just have the patient decide. Obviously speaking in generalities, I do not think the study was understood by must people in the way the authors meant it, and it took multiple readings to actually figure out what I could take away for myself when it first came out. I did not see that this study actually changed practice to a significant degree.

LS

When I heard and read that laparoscopic surgery was not noninferior to open surgery or that the trial was inconclusive regarding the noninferiority of laparoscopic surgery, these were not intuitive concepts.

MD

When both studies were released, my thought process was pretty similar. I distinctly recall reviewing the ACOSOG trial during a journal club session while I was a resident. Upon closer examination of the study details, it became evident that the findings leaned more toward being inconclusive rather than definitive, raising concerns about the oncologic safety of laparoscopy in rectal cancer. I would say that when I was in training and the trial results were published, they did not produce a significant change in clinical practice with the attendings I was working with. Conversely, the ROLARR trial essentially affirmed the safety of robotic surgery but fell short of demonstrating a clear superiority of the technique over laparoscopy, which sparked controversy over whether the investment in robotic technology was warranted. Nonetheless, there was generally less uncertainty regarding the safety and efficacy of robotic surgery compared to laparoscopy in my opinion.

LS

The trial did change my practice at the time because I became disillusioned with the idea of doing laparoscopic surgery for rectal cancer. I had attended meetings, and I had seen videos and talked to surgeons who had told me that it was easier to dissect the pelvis laparoscopically than with open technique. When doing laparoscopic surgery, I did not feel that way. I felt like I could do it safely, and the literature on colon cancer had indicated recovery advantages associated with laparoscopic surgery; therefore, I embraced the trial and I put patients in the trial, waiting for its results. But I also realized in going to trial meetings that the majority of the investigators were very experienced in laparoscopic surgery. My impression was that as a group, we were not approaching the trial with the equipoise that for example a medical oncology group would have in approaching a study comparing 2 chemotherapy regimens. As surgeons, we tend to be very invested in what we do, which can include laparoscopic surgery. We learned it, we went through the learning curve of it, and we tend to believe in it as an advantage for our patients so that it is more difficult to have equipoise when reading the unexpected results of a trial and just change practice. I came into the trial thinking that laparoscopic surgery could provide patient advantages, but I felt that visualization remained difficult. I do not mean to suggest that an open operation is easy, but it did not seem like laparoscopy was making it much easier. After the trial was published I came to the conclusion that if the patient is an obese male with mid or low rectal cancer, I am not going to do his operation laparoscopically anymore, so I started doing more open surgery as a result of the trial. Given my disillusionment with laparoscopic proctectomy, I also became interested in robotic surgery. There was this known issue of higher costs to face, but at the same time, I thought this could be the technique which could make a rectal dissection in a difficult pelvis a little easier. Not easy, but a little easier. I felt I could still do laparoscopic surgery in some of the patients who were not included in the trial, for example, recto-sigmoid cancers, high rectal cancer, earlier disease, leaner patients, women with wider pelvis, etc., and they can do very well and have both an oncologically adequate operation and the recovery advantages of laparoscopic surgery. With respect to the oncologic outcomes, I was not very worried that laparoscopic proctectomy was inherently a worse oncologic operation, I rather felt that setting up the composite pathologic outcome was an ambitious target to achieve. I am pleased that subsequent followup studies have not indicated oncologic differences between the 2 techniques.

AM

I agree with much of what has been said regarding the confusion and conflicting opinions regarding laparoscopic surgery after the publication of this study.

The follow-up report on oncologic outcomes, from this patient cohort, published in Annals of Surgery in 2019 showed similar rates of disease-free survival, locoregional recurrence, and distant recurrence which many held up as evidence of laparoscopic surgery being equivalent to open. However, this trial was not powered to detect these longer-term oncologic outcomes. Thus, at least at the time of this study, the jury was still out on oncologic outcomes of laparoscopy compared to open surgery.

My opinion about the modality used for rectal cancer surgery is that it depends on the individual surgeon. With the technical demands of TME, we must ensure as surgeons that the critical outcome that we wish to optimize is oncologic control, and so the surgeon should choose the modality (open, laparoscopic, or robotic) that they feel can give them the greatest likelihood of achieving an appropriate resection and a complete TME.

Immunotherapy for Locally Advanced Rectal Cancer

19

Cercek A, Lumish M, Sinopoli J, Weiss J, et al. PD-1 blockade in mismatch repair-deficient, locally advanced rectal cancer. N Engl J Med. 2022;386(25):2363–76.

Abstract

Background: Neoadjuvant chemotherapy and radiation followed by surgical resection of the rectum is a standard treatment for locally advanced rectal cancer. A subset of rectal cancer is caused by a deficiency in mismatch repair. Because mismatch repair-deficient colorectal cancer is responsive to programmed death 1 (PD-1) blockade in the context of metastatic disease, it was hypothesized that checkpoint blockade could be effective in patients with mismatch repair-deficient, locally advanced rectal cancer.

Methods: We initiated a prospective phase 2 study in which single-agent dostarlimab, an anti-PD-1 monoclonal antibody, was administered every 3 weeks for 6 months in patients with mismatch repair-deficient stage II or III rectal adenocarcinoma. This treatment was to be followed by standard chemoradiotherapy and surgery. Patients who had a clinical complete response after completion of dostarlimab therapy would proceed without chemoradiotherapy and surgery. The primary endpoints are sustained clinical complete response 12 months after completion of dostarlimab therapy or pathological complete response after completion of dostarlimab therapy with or without chemoradiotherapy and overall response to neoadjuvant dostarlimab therapy with or without chemoradiotherapy.

Results: A total of 12 patients have completed treatment with dostarlimab and have undergone at least 6 months of follow-up. All 12 patients (100%; 95% confidence interval, 74–100) had a clinical complete response, with no evidence of tumor on magnetic resonance imaging, 18F-fluorodeoxyglucose-positron-emission tomography, endoscopic evaluation, digital rectal examination, or biopsy. At the time of this report, no patients had received chemoradiotherapy or undergone surgery, and no cases of progression or recurrence had been reported during follow-up (range, 6–25 months). No adverse events of grade 3 or higher have been reported.

Conclusions: Mismatch repair-deficient, locally advanced rectal cancer was highly sensitive to single-agent PD-1 blockade. Longer follow-up is needed to assess the duration of response.

DC

This is another landmark study in the evolution of rectal cancer treatment. Admittedly, this is only applicable to rectal cancers that are mismatch repair-deficient (MMR-D), somewhere between 2 and 10% of all rectal cancers [1, 2]. This includes the Lynch syndrome variants and the much more common, sporadic MMR-D rectal cancers. It is clear that these cancers do behave differently, as MMR-Ds are not sensitive to treatment with 5-fluorouracil, and lymphocytic infiltration is more common and tends to be of lower pathological stage [2].

Previous studies in metastatic, MMR-D rectal cancer have shown survival benefits with the use of pembrolizumab, a programmed death 1 (PD-1) inhibitor. This study intended to have an arm that had pembrolizumab only and another that had pembrolizumab, chemoradiation, and then surgery. However, because all 12 included patients who received pembrolizumab had a sustained clinical response (by digital rectal examination, endoscopy, and MRI) 1 year after the start of the trial, the other arm could not be recruited. Though the study is reported to have recruited both stage II and III patients, only one stage II patient was recruited, the remainder stage III. There is one study that was able to enroll 5/44 patients with MMR-D locally advanced cancer (the rest 39 MMR-normal) which underwent chemoradiotherapy, then pembrolizumab, and then resection. All patients underwent the same treatment, but only the MMR-D patients had 100% relapse-free survival at 3 years (compared to 80%) [3, 4]. There has been no shortage of enthusiasm for using PDL-1 inhibitors in colorectal cancer, and in a recent study, 68% of the colon cancer patients treated with 2 PD-1 inhibitors had a complete pathological response [5]. Though analyzing the rationale for dual PD-1 inhibitor in colon cancers is beyond the scope of this communication, suffice it to say that PD-1 inhibitors will be universally used in all MMR-D rectal cancers, with great expectations of disease-free survival (though little data on 5-year disease-free survival exists of yet). It is hard to believe that such a small study made such a great impact, but the nearly 100% reproducibility of their findings is hard to ignore.

References

1. Alatise OI, Knapp GC, Sharma A, et al. Molecular and phenotypic profiling of colorectal cancer patients in West Africa reveals biological insights. Nat Commun. 2021;12:6821.
2. Farchoukh LF, Celebrezze J, Medich D, et al. DNA mismatch repair-deficient rectal cancer is frequently associated with Lynch syndrome and with poor response to neoadjuvant therapy. Am J Surg Pathol. 2022;46:1260–8.
3. Vilar E, Gruber S. Microsatellite instability in colorectal cancer—the stable evidence. Nat Rev. Clin Oncol. 2010;7:153–62. https://doi.org/10.1038/nrclinonc.2009.237
4. Tsukada Y, Bando H, Inamori K, et al. Three-year outcomes of preoperative chemoradiotherapy plus nivolumab in microsatellite stable and microsatellite instability-high locally advanced rectal cancer. Br J Cancer. 2024;131(2):283–9.
5. Chalabi M, Verschoor YL, Batista Tan P, et al. Neoadjuvant immunotherapy in locally advanced mismatch repair–deficient colon cancer. N Engl J Med. 2024;390:1949–58.

Discussion

DC

This study influenced greatly how we treat mismatch repair deficient rectal cancers. Using this PD-1 inhibitor (now multiple drugs within this class) essentially melts cancers away, at least these specific rectal cancers. It is hard to argue with their findings, especially since they have been reproduced. I do not know for sure if we have solid 5-year outcomes, but that will be interesting to see, and I am very optimistic.

LS

The update to this trial waspresented at the latest ASCO (Cercek, J Clin Oncol 42, 2024 (suppl 17; abstr LBA3512)) and confirmed sustained response after a median follow-up of 29 months. I agree that we need to wait for the 5-year outcomes. I feel that after such a dramatic result, the question becomes to which extent we should approach all MMR-D colorectal cancers with PD-1 blockade as first-line treatment and utilize surgery only as salvage treatment. This would include, for example, colon cancers that are amenable to resection, rather than metastatic disease of locally advanced rectal cancers, which was the population of this particular study. An important question is also the prevention of metachronous cancers especially in Lynch syndrome, and there is a subpopulation of patients with MMR-D cancer in the background of inflammatory bowel disease in whom the role of PD-1 inhibitors would make sense, but we do not have lots of data about it. A particular finding which constitutes a challenge in MMR-D cancers after PD-1 inhibitor treatment is a residual mass visible radiologically associated with pathologic complete response after resection. This is a known phenomenon after chemo(radio)therapy in MMR proficient tumors but seems to be more pronounced in the MMR-D subpopulation. I feel future investigations should focus on methods to identify patients who have a complete treatment response despite a residual radiological mass and still could be saved from surgery.

MD

Yes, I was going to echo that. We looked at our own data, we looked at about seven patients that we had treated with PD-1 inhibitors, and they seem to use pembrolizumab more frequently than dostarlimab. In our series, none of them had radiographically complete responses. And many of them, four of them, had undergone major surgical procedures including pelvic exenteration, abdominoperineal resection, etc., and four of them had complete pathologic responses despite large, bulky tumors being seen on MRI. I feel that with these types of tumors, the disconnect between radiographic findings and pathologic findings is more enhanced in that the tumors look quite bulky on MRI but then end up having a complete pathologic response, whereas in the MSI stable tumors, generally, if there is a big, bulky tumor, there's still disease in the pathologic specimen. Therefore, I think that the study is exciting with regard to this patient population in terms of avoiding radiation and surgery, but we still have some ways to go with regard to determining or being able to capture those patients who don't have a radiographic response, but still have a complete pathologic response like you were saying. This could be better imaging or perhaps blood testing looking for tumor markers, etc. I think that will be the next step in these types of tumors.

DC

So, it is more that radiologic findings indicate that there could be a tumor, but when this is excised and examined pathologically, it is not. Is that correct?

MD

Yes, and when I looked at the actual MRIs, it is not like subtle findings. Possibly, there is something like when we are talking about a near-complete response, they look like big mucinous tumors that are even invading other structures, but then all that tumor is actually tissue without any disease. It is interesting they do not really note that in this study, but when we looked at our data, a lot of the patients were in that situation. And a lot of other retrospective reviews and other institutions also indicate that the MRI technology does not have sufficient specificity to tell us whether it is scar or tumor, not yet at least.

AM

Agree, this is clearly a significant milestone in the treatment of colorectal cancer. The issues you speak of with regard to knowing which patients have truly achieved pathologic complete response on PD-1 blockade are analogous to the problems we have in predicting this in complete clinical responders in general. Our testing, whether MRI imaging, blood, or others, is not of sufficient resolution yet to accurately determine this 100% of the time. Furthermore, MRI technology and protocol techniques are very variable, and at least in the United States, insufficient standards exist which are not uniform wherever the patient goes.

Also, while this study demonstrated a 100% response rate, this has not always been seen in practice, and so it is also necessary to temper expectations of patients.

Surgery for Locally Recurrent Rectal Cancer

20

van Kessel CS, Solomon MJ. Understanding the philosophy, anatomy, and surgery of the extra-TME plane of locally advanced and locally recurrent rectal cancer; single institution experience with international benchmarking. Cancers (Basel). 2022;14(20):5058.

Abstract

Objective: To assess the results of multimodality therapy for patients with recurrent rectal cancer and to analyze factors predictive of curative resection and prognostic for overall survival.

Summary of Background Data: Locally recurrent rectal cancer is a difficult clinical problem, and radical treatment options with curative intent are not generally accepted.

Methods: A total of 394 patients underwent surgical exploration for recurrent rectal cancer. Ninety were found to have unresectable local or extrapelvic disease and 304 underwent resection of the recurrence. The latter patients were prospectively followed to determine long-term survival and factors influencing survival.

Results: Overall 5-year survival was 25%. Curative, negative resection margins were obtained in 45% of patients; in these patients, a 5-year survival of 37% was achieved, compared to 16% ($P < 0.001$) in patients with either microscopic or gross residual disease. In a logistic regression analysis, initial surgery with end-colostomy and symptomatic pain (both univariate) and increasing number of sites of the recurrent tumor fixation in the pelvis (multivariate) were associated with palliative surgery. Overall survival was significantly decreased for symptomatic pain ($P < 0.001$) and more than one fixation ($P = 0.029$). Survival following extended resection of adjacent organs was not different from limited resection (28% vs. 21%, $P = 0.11$). Patient demographics and factors related to the initial rectal cancer did not affect outcome. Perioperative mortality was only 0.3%, but significant morbidity occurred in 26% of patients, with pelvic abscess being the most common complication.

Conclusions: This study demonstrates that many patients with locally recurrent rectal cancer can be resected with negative margins. Long-term survival can be achieved, especially for patients with no symptoms and minimal fixation of the recurrence in the pelvis, provided no gross residual disease remains.

DC

This review comes from a well-respected group with a wealth of experience in treating recurrent rectal cancers and a publication track record to prove their well-deserved place as experts in the field. At the very heart of this paper lies the question of whether we—as a specialty, or at least those of us who treat recurrent rectal cancer—are veering away from extensive resections and toward using more chemotherapy or radiotherapy. This was the report's underlying premise.

The data used to illustrate this dichotomy is obtained from their own institutional experience at the Royal Prince Alfred Hospital (RPA) and the PelvEx Collaborative. "The PelvEx Collaborative is an international collaborative group involving over 140 units across five continents, with the aim to examine outcomes for patients who have had pelvic exenterative surgery."—from their own website [1].

There are three principal data-driven observations that support this report's underlying premise: (1) The PelvEx collaborative uses perioperative radiation more frequently, (2) the R0 rate is higher in the RPA group (compared to the PelvEx group), and 3. the median overall survival (OS) rate is higher in the RPA group. It is especially worth mentioning that the difference here is especially stark, with a mean OS of 95 months (almost 8 years) in the

RPA group and 37 months (3 years) in the PelvEx group. Given the ongoing enrollment of this multinational group, one would not expect a median follow-up longer than 3 years. Thus, this comparison is difficult to interpret because of this limitation. An OS of mid-70 to mid-80s at 2 years is considered high, and it is rare to see it past mid-40s at 5 years [2, 3]. Much of the rest of the report focuses on technical aspects of the surgery, systematic presentation and description no doubt helpful to many readers.

While it is true that the patients presented here from the PelvEx group received more chemoradiation, it does not necessarily follow that this was done at the expense of a less radical resection. In fact, their own publication in 2019 indicates the exact opposite [4]. The lower R0 rate in the PelvEx group is not unexpected given that the data comes from many centers in multiple countries spread across multiple continents. One would expect that the treatment will inherently have some heterogeneity, though multiple efforts have been made to increase collaboration and homogeneity.

The authors are absolutely right in their assertion that R0 must be achieved whenever possible, and to do that, a systematic approach must be employed in a specialist center within a group of experienced multidisciplinary doctors, and the surgery performed by experienced surgeons. This however would be the same thing any other surgeon performing these surgeries would say, and I do not think that an emphasis on utilization of perioperative radiation and chemotherapy when indicated necessarily comes at the expense of an adequate resection. They are used as they are intended, adjuvants, not replacements of excellent technique. A seminal study at another institution with extensive experience in treating recurrent and locally advanced rectal cancer has more than two decades ago successfully shown that R0 resection can result in long-term survival in those patients with minimal fixation (an alternative and probably more helpful criteria of preoperatively predicting tumor resectability). Moreover, they do show that preoperative chemoradiation and intraoperative radiation are useful even in those patients who have advanced disease [5]. There is a lot of contemporary data regarding the advantages of proper utilization of chemotherapy and radiation (both external beam and internal) in this setting, and that discussion is beyond the scope of this communication.

References

1. PelvEx Collaborative website. https://www.pelvex.org. Accessed 3 Nov 2023.
2. Gould LE, Pring ET, Drami I, Moorghen M, Naghibi M, Jenkins JT, Steele CW, Roxburgh CS. A systematic review of the pathological determinants of outcome following resection by pelvic exenteration of locally advanced and locally recurrent rectal cancer. Int J Surg. 2022;104:106738. https://doi.org/10.1016/j.ijsu.2022.106738. Epub 2022 Jul 1. PMID: 35781038.
3. Colibaseanu DT, Dozois EJ, Mathis KL, et al. Extended sacropelvic resection for locally recurrent rectal cancer: can it be done safely and with good oncologic outcomes? Dis Colon Rectum 2014;57:47–55. https://doi.org/10.1097/DCR.000000000000001.
4. PelvEx Collaborative. Changing outcomes following pelvic exenteration for locally advanced and recurrent rectal cancer. BJS Open. 2019;3(4):516–20. doi: 10.1002/bjs5.50153. PMID: 31388644; PMCID: PMC6677093.
5. Hahnloser D, Nelson H, Gunderson LL, Hassan I, Haddock MG, O'Connell MJ, Cha S, Sargent DJ, Horgan A. Curative potential of multimodality therapy for locally recurrent rectal cancer. Ann Surg. 2003;237(4):502–8. doi: https://doi.org/10.1097/01.SLA.0000059972.90598.5F. PMID: 12677146; PMCID: PMC1514480.

Discussion

DC

This paper is from a group with the experience to say a lot about this topic. This is an interesting paper that does multiple things. It describes a systematic approach to these tumors, discusses the importance of R0 resection, and warns against what they perceive as deviations from that R0 pursuit. It is absolutely true that these surgeries are beasts to perform in most cases, and even with R0 resection, and even with best preoperative imaging, and demonstrative lack of metastatic disease, too many of these patients still ultimately die from metastatic disease. So then, in that sense, we must do everything we can to obtain R0 both by careful selection of the patients and operative technique and expertise.

And I think the PelvEx group would agree with everything said here, so I think that is where the paper and I part ways, because I do not know of a single colorectal surgeon or surgeon oncologist who would argue that radiation and chemotherapy are anything other than adjuncts to an R0 resection.... in an ideal world. That world does not exist, so you would expect that in a heterogenous group, across multiple institutions and countries, with many surgeons, a bigger proportion of the surgeries will have R1 resections. Nothing about that is surprising. Though beyond the scope of this discussion, the merits of adjuvant therapy (radiation and/or chemotherapy) in R1 disease have been well established. This is another excellent addition to their already significant contribution to this difficult topic, without a doubt.

MD

I thought it was a great review and agree that toward the end of the paper, when they are going over their techniques for recurrent or advanced disease in different compartments, I thought that was excellent. And they obviously are very well known and have a lot of experience. And they have seen that their patients are doing better with time as they have revised their practice. Overall, what I got from this, though, was that they are, in general, very aggressive with regard to their resection and what they are doing. If you look at the numbers, the amount of sacrectomy that they are doing is 58.9% vs. 20.3% in the Pelvex group. Overall, I think that the point of this paper is to say that, as you were saying, we should not rely on neoadjuvant radiation, and chemotherapy has a place, but it does not supplant the need for a large operation to obtain that R0 margin because that is so critical with regard to local recurrence and recurrence-free survival.

LS

I agree with you all. This is impressive, particularly in the description of the techniques, especially for the anterior compartment. I certainly do not have the experience of Michael Solomon and this group. I have done sacrectomy procedures, always in collaboration with neurosurgery or orthopedic surgery, but never done anterior resection of pubic rami and a portion of the symphysis, so I am very impressed by that part. I think philosophically I feel that we should view available treatments as complementary, and I think there is no debate that we should not conceive the use of chemotherapy and radiotherapy as true alternatives to surgery. I think that, however, we should continue exploring the avenues where chemotherapy and radiotherapy, either in the neoadjuvant, intraoperative, and/or postoperative settings can contribute to optimal oncologic outcomes. We should try and establish the specific and ideal situations where these treatments play a role. And I cannot understand if these are used at all in the Authors' institution. I could not understand to which extent it was cultural aversion vs. lack of institutional support from those services for these complex cases. Having said that, I do admire the work that this unit has done. I do respect the justifiable pride in presenting very good oncologic data when compared to the combined data of a consortium of multiple institutions. I think that among patients with locally recurrent rectal cancer, there is a subgroup of patients with lesions where it can be difficult to predict based on imaging if an R0 resection is possible, and ultimately, the surgical result could be an R1 resection. I feel that if patients are motivated, are in good general condition, and have completed chemotherapy and external beam radiotherapy as indicated, it is worthwhile to proceed with surgery understanding that the pursuit of an R0 resection might still result in R1 resection. In individual cases, this might also lead to palliative benefit, for example, in relieving patients from local symptoms.

Laparoscopic vs. Open Colectomy for Colon Cancer

21

Clinical Outcomes of Surgical Therapy Study Group; Nelson H, Sargent DJ, Wieand HS, Fleshman J, Anvari M, Stryker SJ, Beart RW Jr., Hellinger M, Flanagan R Jr., Peters W, Ota D. A comparison of laparoscopically assisted and open colectomy for colon cancer. N Engl J Med. 2004;350(20):2050–9.

Abstract

Background: Minimally invasive, laparoscopically assisted surgery was first considered in 1990 for patients undergoing colectomy for cancer. Concern that this approach would compromise survival by failing to achieve a proper oncologic resection or adequate staging or by altering patterns of recurrence (based on frequent reports of tumor recurrences within surgical wounds) prompted a controlled trial evaluation.

Methods: We conducted a noninferiority trial at 48 institutions and randomly assigned 872 patients with adenocarcinoma of the colon to undergo open or laparoscopically assisted colectomy performed by credentialed surgeons. The median follow-up was 4.4 years. The primary endpoint was the time to tumor recurrence.

Results: At 3 years, the rates of recurrence were similar in the two groups: 16% among patients in the group that underwent laparoscopically assisted surgery and 18% among patients in the open-colectomy group (two-sided $P = 0.32$; hazard ratio for recurrence, 0.86; 95% confidence interval, 0.63–1.17). Recurrence

© The Author(s), under exclusive license to Springer Nature Switzerland AG 2025

D. Colibaseanu et al., *Essential Articles in Colorectal Surgery*,
https://doi.org/10.1007/978-3-031-77745-5_21

rates in surgical wounds were less than 1% in both groups ($P = 0.50$). The overall survival rate at 3 years was also very similar in the two groups (86% in the laparoscopic-surgery group and 85% in the open-colectomy group; $P = 0.51$; hazard ratio for death in the laparoscopic-surgery group, 0.91; 95% confidence interval, 0.68–1.21), with no significant difference between groups in the time to recurrence or overall survival for patients with any stage of cancer. Perioperative recovery was faster in the laparoscopic-surgery group than in the open-colectomy group, as reflected by a shorter median hospital stay (5 days vs. 6 days, $P < 0.001$) and briefer use of parenteral narcotics (3 days vs. 4 days, $P < 0.001$) and oral analgesics (1 day vs. 2 days, $P = 0.02$). The rates of intraoperative complications, 30-day postoperative mortality, complications at discharge and 60 days, hospital readmission, and reoperation were very similar between groups.

Conclusions: In this multi-institutional study, the rates of recurrent cancer were similar after laparoscopically assisted colectomy and open colectomy, suggesting that the laparoscopic approach is an acceptable alternative to open surgery for colon cancer.

LS

This is a fundamental article which influenced the advent of laparoscopic surgery for colon cancer in the United States and in the world. The noninferiority study design was specifically suited to demonstrate that laparoscopic surgery was at least comparable to open colectomy without attempting to demonstrate improved outcomes. However, the postoperative use of parenteral narcotics was significantly reduced, and the hospital stay was significantly shorter after laparoscopic surgery. These advantages have become often reported following minimally invasive surgery when compared to open surgery for a variety of other conditions. The selection of surgeons participating in this trial required a credentialing procedure where the surgeons needed to demonstrate they had performed at least 20 laparoscopically assisted colorectal operations and also had to submit a video of one of their laparoscopic colonic resections which was reviewed to confirm that the conduct of the operation was consistent with the accepted principles of oncologic surgery. It is notable that 21% of the cases were converted to open colectomy and still kept in the laparoscopic group in an intent-to-treat analysis, which still allowed for a statistically significant difference in recovery parameters. A clinical concern which was widely debated at the time and almost derailed the trial was the possibility of increased rate of tumor recurrence at the level of the extraction site or other port sites following laparoscopic colectomy [1]. Ultimately, the issue of wound recurrence lost traction as this was demonstrated to be a possible but very rare event, occurring after both laparoscopic and open surgery. Several retrospective series, prospective randomized trials conducted elsewhere in the world, and follow-up studies did not confirm any alarming increase in the incidence of wound recurrences while reaffirming the recovery advantages following laparoscopic surgery [2–4]. I feel it is safe to say that the problem of wound recurrence following minimally invasive surgery is no longer widely debated today. In the 20 years following the publication of this trial, laparoscopic colectomy has been widely accepted, while significant progress has continued in minimally invasive surgery including the widespread adoption of enhanced recovery protocols and the introduction of robotic surgery. Probably, the hospital stay following minimally invasive colectomy at this time and age would be even shorter, and the conversion rate would be lower than in the COST trial. With the advent of robotic surgery, the debate has shifted on whether intracorporeal anastomosis is associated with further acceleration of postoperative recovery [5]. While some data indicate that robotic surgery provides additional advantages compared with laparoscopic surgery, the debate remains open. However, an imminent prospective randomized trial addressing this question with a scope and magnitude comparable to that of the COST trial remains unlikely.

References

1. Berends FJ, Kazemier G, Bonjer HJ, Lange JF. Subcutaneous metastases after laparoscopic colectomy. Lancet. 1994;344(8914):58.

2. Veldkamp R, Kuhry E, Hop WC, Jeekel J, Kazemier G, Bonjer HJ, Haglind E, Påhlman L, Cuesta MA, Msika S, Morino M, Lacy AM; COlon cancer Laparoscopic or Open Resection Study Group (COLOR). Laparoscopic surgery versus open surgery for colon cancer: short-term outcomes of a randomised trial. Lancet Oncol. 2005;6(7):477–84.
3. Hewett PJ, Allardyce RA, Bagshaw PF, Frampton CM, Frizelle FA, Rieger NA, Smith JS, Solomon MJ, Stephens JH, Stevenson AR. Short-term outcomes of the Australasian randomized clinical study comparing laparoscopic and conventional open surgical treatments for colon cancer: the ALCCaS trial. Ann Surg. 2008;248(5):728–38.
4. Fleshman J, Sargent DJ, Green E, Anvari M, Stryker SJ, Beart RW Jr., Hellinger M, Flanagan R Jr., Peters W, Nelson H; Clinical Outcomes of Surgical Therapy Study Group. Laparoscopic colectomy for cancer is not inferior to open surgery based on 5-year data from the COST Study Group trial. Ann Surg. 2007;246(4):655–62; discussion 662–4.
5. Cleary RK, Silviera M, Reidy TJ, McCormick J, Johnson CS, Sylla P, Cannon J, Lujan H, Kassir A, Landmann R, Gaertner W, Lee E, Bastawrous A, Bardakcioglu O, Pandey S, Attaluri V, Bernstein M, Obias V, Franklin ME Jr., Pigazzi A. Intracorporeal and extracorporeal anastomosis for robotic-assisted and laparoscopic right colectomy: short-term outcomes of a multi-center prospective trial. Surg Endosc. 2022;36(6):4349–58.

Discussion

DC

This is a trial headed by Dr. Heidi Nelson. This trial was a noninferiority trial, but as opposed to more contemporary noninferiority trials, the primary endpoint was tumor recurrence, not adjuncts to oncologic outcomes. This was a multi-institution study, excellently designed, with 428 patients randomized in the open group and 435 in the laparoscopic group. At the end of the study with a follow-up time of 4.4 years, the investigators found a similar recurrence and overall survival, but because of the design and power of the study, the statistically supported conclusion was that the laparoscopic group was noninferior. In other words, it was an oncologically acceptable alternative to open surgery for colon cancer. It had other perioperative benefits that made the technique superior to the open approach, but at the very least, they showed that there was no oncologic detriment to using this newer technique.

MD

Yes, this is another noninferiority study. Not necessarily looking if laparoscopic surgery was superior to open. But I do agree this was a landmark study at the time, accepting laparoscopic surgery for the treatment of colon cancer, and it led the way to the rectal cancer studies, which I know we talked a lot about separately. What was interesting was that their conversion rate was 21% and patients converted to open were all kept in the same laparoscopic arm, and they still were associated with significant advantages with regard to length of stay. I think the one caveat with this study is that they excluded locally advanced tumors, so this trial did not address the treatment of larger, bulkier tumors. With robotic surgery, I think now we are pushing the envelope more and more with the types of tumors we are treating. I think this also speaks to the FOxTROT trial and the role of neoadjuvant chemotherapy for some of these tumors. And I think now the conversation revolves more around the role of robotic surgery vs. laparoscopic and if there are any advantages with that and also looking at intracorporeal anastomosis.

LS

I think the noninferiority trial was very useful in this particular situation, and this was the template which was used by the subsequent rectal cancer studies which have generated so many questions, but in this particular trial, it did work very well. I am not a statistician, and I am not experienced in the design of large trials, but I know that a noninferiority design requires fewer patients and, therefore, less effort and less expenses than a superiority trial, everything else being equal. In this particular case, even though a formal superiority trial could not be determined based on the outcomes of interest, when looking at outcomes, as Michelle pointed out, particularly recovery parameters, there is an obvious advantage in favor of laparoscopy. This is the trial that unleashed the use of laparoscopy for colon cancer, so it remains a landmark trial. One question that is fascinating to me is why for the advent of robotic surgery we do not need a similar trial of laparoscopic vs. robotic surgery for colon cancer and why the situation seems to be so different from that time to the point that there seems to be no impetus to create a trial.

MD

Yes, ideally.

DC

The same method or similar method was applied to rectal cancer, as another noninferiority trial (talking about Z6051), but not exactly, at least not to measured outcomes. Then, the results were confusing for a lot of people, and many frankly ignored the trial. I mean, if the trial said that we could not say that laparoscopic proctectomies are an acceptable alternative (or failed to meet noninferiority), then the logical outcome should have been that laparoscopic proctectomies in the US stopped. Did that happen? No, not even close. Why? Because there were issues with the trial design that some recognized, and frankly, it is not easy to actually figure out what a noninferiority trial shows when it fails to show noninferiority. When we talked about the Z6051 noninferiority trial, I brought up that there was a study showing that many people just straight up misinterpret the trials… even in their publications referencing these trials. Others just do not know what to make of the results. In part, because of the design of the trials, in part because of the general methodologic lack of expertise in this area on the part of the readers, me included.

Of course, at least in the US, the patients have a big say in what we do, and industry has its influence too, so probably all those forces resulted in Z6051 largely being ignored (with a few exceptions) as opposed to the COST trial.

MD

Our trials are not perfect.

Neoadjuvant Chemotherapy for Locally Advanced Colon Cancer

22

Morton D, Seymour M, Magill L, Handley K, Glasbey J, Glimelius B, Palmer A, Seligmann J, Laurberg S, Murakami K, West N, Quirke P, Gray R; FOxTROT Collaborative Group. Preoperative chemotherapy for operable colon cancer: mature results of an international randomized controlled trial. J Clin Oncol. 2023;41(8):1541–52.

Abstract

Purpose: Neoadjuvant chemotherapy (NAC) has potential advantages over standard postoperative chemotherapy for locally advanced colon cancer but requires formal evaluation.

Methods: Patients with radiologically staged T3-4, N0-2, M0 colon cancer were randomly allocated (2:1) to 6 weeks oxaliplatin–fluoropyrimidine preoperatively plus 18 postoperatively (NAC group) or 24 weeks postoperatively (control group). Patients with RAS-wild-type tumors could also be randomly assigned 1:1 to receive panitumumab or not during NAC. The primary endpoint was residual disease or recurrence within 2 years. Secondary outcomes included surgical morbidity, histopathologic stage, regression grade, completeness of resection, and cause-specific mortality. Log-rank analyses were performed by intention-to-treat.

Results: Of 699 patients allocated to NAC, 674 (96%) started and 606 (87%) completed NAC. In total, 686 of 699 (98.1%) NAC

© The Author(s), under exclusive license to Springer Nature Switzerland AG 2025
D. Colibaseanu et al., *Essential Articles in Colorectal Surgery*,
https://doi.org/10.1007/978-3-031-77745-5_22

patients and 351 of 354 (99.2%) control patients underwent surgery. Thirty patients (4.3%) allocated to NAC developed obstructive symptoms requiring expedited surgery, but there were fewer serious postoperative complications with NAC than with control. NAC produced marked T and N downstaging and histologic tumor regression (all $P < 0.001$). Resection was more often histopathologically complete: 94% (648/686) versus 89% (311/351), $P < 0.001$. Fewer NAC than control patients had residual or recurrent disease within 2 years (16.9% [118/699] vs. 21.5% [76/354]; rate ratio, 0.72 [95% CI, 0.54–0.98]; $P = 0.037$). Tumor regression correlated strongly with freedom from recurrence. Panitumumab did not enhance the benefit from NAC. Little benefit from NAC was seen in mismatch repair-deficient tumors.

Conclusion: Six weeks of preoperative oxaliplatin-fluoropyrimidine chemotherapy for operable colon cancer can be delivered safely, without increasing perioperative morbidity. This chemotherapy regimen, when given preoperatively, produces marked histopathologic downstaging, fewer incomplete resections, and better 2-year disease control. Histologic regression after NAC is a strong predictor of lower postoperative recurrence risk so has potential use as a guide for postoperative therapy. Six weeks of NAC should be considered as a treatment option for locally advanced colon cancer.

LS

This is the quintessential trial which has established the role of neoadjuvant chemotherapy in locally advanced colon cancer. It has changed our practice, and it is here to stay. The study was based on 85 different surgical centers, and therefore, I feel that its results can be generalized. The definition of locally advanced colon cancer was cT3-4 M0 based on CT assessment and changed after the pilot phase of the study and ended up including patients who had a cT3 tumor extending beyond the colonic wall by at least 1 mm vs. the initial 5 mm. The selection criteria did not attempt to select patients based on any regional lymph node characteristics. The trial data on toxicity and lack of disease progression during neoadjuvant treatment are reassuring. A corollary study on post hoc data investigated the 4.3% proportion of patients who experienced bowel obstruction requiring urgent surgery during the course of neoadjuvant chemotherapy leading to a higher rate of R1 resections. The factors associated with the risk of bowel obstruction during neoadjuvant chemotherapy were inability to pass the endoscope at the time of initial diagnosis or obstructing cancers based on imaging [1], which is not surprising. This remains a low rate considering that alternatively, upfront surgery would be associated with significant morbidity from the excision of often large tumors that could be invading adjacent organs. This is a subgroup of patients which could be counseled about these risks, but I would not necessarily consider these features as absolute contraindications to neoadjuvant chemotherapy. Encouraging results from neoadjuvant chemotherapy use have been replicated in the PRODIGE 22 trial in France [2] and elsewhere. In a meta-analysis of 7 studies including a total of 2120 patients, neoadjuvant chemotherapy was associated with increased survival and disease-free survival when compared with initial surgery without any increase in complications at the time of surgery. In addition, neoadjuvant chemotherapy was associated with a lower risk of incomplete resection [3]. Skeptics on the use of neoadjuvant chemotherapy in locally advanced colon cancer have pointed out the risk of overtreatment given the limitation in the accuracy of CT scans. The reported overtreatment rate in the control group of the FOxTROT trial based on the comparison between pathologic staging and preoperative CT staging was 24%. Assuming a similar rate of overtreatment in the neoadjuvant chemotherapy group, this might be at least in part a reason explaining the decreased disease recurrence rates associated with the neoadjuvant treatment group. It is difficult to assess the intrinsic advantage of neoadjuvant vs. upfront surgery if we consider for example a cT3 lesion marginally extending beyond the colonic wall. However, the FOxTROT trial publication corroborates neoadjuvant chemotherapy as a safe and feasible option at least for those difficult colonic tumors which are bulky and/or invade adjacent structures on CT scan. Without these data, the idea of reducing the burden of disease with neoadjuvant chemotherapy would seem logical, but it might have been impractical to convince our oncology colleagues to start chemotherapy with their inherent toxicity risks without solid supportive data. Future studies will focus on neoadjuvant chemotherapy in the elderly (FOxTROT 2) and different chemotherapy agent combinations (FOxTROT 3) [4].

References

1. Glasbey J; FOxTROT Collaborating Group. Risk of bowel obstruction in patients undergoing neoadjuvant chemotherapy for high-risk colon cancer: a nested case-control matched analysis of an international, multi-centre, randomised controlled trial (FOxTROT). Ann Surg. 2024;280(2):283–93.
2. Karoui M, Gallois C, Piessen G, Legoux JL, Barbier E, De Chaisemartin C, Lecaille C, Bouche O, Ammarguellat H, Brunetti F, Prudhomme M, Regimbeau JM, Glehen O, Lievre A, Portier G, Hartwig J, Goujon G, Romain B, Lepage C, Taieb J; for PRODIGE 22 Investigators/Collaborators. Does neoadjuvant FOLFOX chemotherapy improve the prognosis of high-risk Stage II and III colon cancers? Three years' follow-up results of the PRODIGE 22 phase II randomized multicentre trial. Colorectal Dis. 2021;23(6):1357–69.
3. Aliseda D, Arredondo J, Sánchez-Justicia C, Alvarellos A, Rodríguez J, Matos I, Rotellar F, Baixauli J, Pastor C. Survival and safety after neoadjuvant chemotherapy or upfront surgery for locally advanced colon cancer: meta-analysis. Br J Surg. 2024;111(2):znae021.
4. Platt JR, Williams CJM, Craig Z, Cairns DA, Glasbey JC, Morton D, Seligmann J. Personalizing neoadjuvant chemotherapy for locally advanced colon cancer: protocols for the international phase III FOxTROT2 and FOxTROT3 randomized controlled trials. Colorectal Dis. 2023;25(3):357–66. Epub 2023 Feb 15. PMID: 36710525.

Discussion

AM

Some of the concerns when FOxTROT was first published were that the concept was to give neoadjuvant chemotherapy for locally advanced colon cancer to, presumably, optimally downstage the tumor and improve outcomes. But when you start looking at the data, I think in the initial publication, nearly or over three-fourths of the patients had less than T4 tumors. And the T4s are the ones that presumably are the most difficult in terms of achieving a complete resection, an R0 reception. The rest were somewhere between pT1 and T3, but N0 disease. And so those were patients that would not necessarily have received chemotherapy anyway, granted the uncertainty of tumor staging determined after patients underwent neoadjuvant chemotherapy. Second, I think the distant recurrence rate is not reported when the thought was to give chemotherapy to decrease micrometastatic disease. My other concern is that the trial utilizes a CT scan to help predict the extent of the disease, and so there is definitely a risk of overtreatment since CT is variable and not necessarily as accurate in determining the true extent of the disease. This is, I think, not a small risk in this population. It's a good trial in that it's a large, randomized trial which puts forth this concept of neoadjuvant treatment, but I just don't know if it's something that we can blanket apply to all patients with what we presume to be locally advanced disease without improved preoperative imaging, maybe Magnetic Resonance (MR), MRs done with a high-quality scanner.

DC

I would agree with all of that. I would say that definitely in this era, where we rely so much on MRI which might not be the "official" imaging standard, but it is nearly so in practice. It is hard to go back to the CT for the purposes of trying to apply this trial's precepts in treating our patients, and I am not sure that the findings apply uniformly to patients that are T1, T2, or T4. Also, we are using MRI so often now that staging and, therefore, treatment decisions are more difficult to interpret from the lens of this trial which uses CT. There is no doubt that this trial is brought up many times during our Tumor Board meetings, and that is valid and useful and represents great work.

MD

I agree with all of that. I think it was a well-done trial, and I think it is most applicable to the obviously T4 tumors that are very bulky or with very big, large nodal disease. But again, as was stated, I think we run the risk of overtreatment in this patient population, specifically with the T3N0 or T2N0 cancers. I thought it was interesting that it seemed like they were still giving adjuvant therapy, despite the pathology results to patients with T3N0 tumors in this trial, which I do not know if they wanted to do that to be consistent, but that was something that just caught my attention when reading through the trial. And though they do show that the 2-year loco-regional recurrence was improved in the neoadjuvant chemotherapy group, again, they did not talk about overall or disease-free survival, which I think they mentioned that the study was not powered for. So again, I think it is applicable to certain situations. But I do not think it necessarily changes overall management in the population that they mentioned, and again, specifically because of our limitations with radiology.

AM

The other thing is that the trial analyzes a prolonged period of chemotherapy, whereas now, really, the standard is shifted after the IDEA trial (Iverson TJ, JCO 2021) to 3 months. For probably most patients or many patients, as opposed to 6 months and so, patients are potentially receiving, at least under the paradigm of FOxTROT, a long period of chemotherapy with a higher risk of toxicity.

LS

I agree with you that it is difficult to test FOxTROT for all patients who, in retrospect, you might say we could have given neoadjuvant instead of adjuvant treatment because they have clinically positive lymph nodes when at best they actually have T3N0 lesions. I think what has changed to me is the perception that it is safe and suitable to give neoadjuvant treatment for large tumors. So, when I am faced with large tumors not necessarily T4s, but, for example, a right colon tumor that extends into the retroperitoneum on CT and I'm not sure if it's attached or if it's close to structures, let's say the duodenum or, if it is associated with visible, large mesocolic lymph nodes. It is not a common situation, but it is a challenging situation where, obviously, we are not sure about the status of the lymph nodes, but they are abnormal on CT scan. I think neoadjuvant chemotherapy is now my preference over doing surgery upfront. And I feel that because of this trial, there is agreement and there is not much of a discussion. You do not need to convince an oncologist about it. In the past, I had the same ideas on the sequence of treatments under the same circumstances, based on the data on downstaging locally advanced disease in rectal cancer, but it was more difficult to convince the oncologists to give neoadjuvant chemotherapy because there was no scientific basis from a well-designed trial. You alluded before to the possibility that MR could be better at staging tumors, and honestly, I do not know the data about it. So far, I would use a CT scan, but if there's new information about the greater accuracy of MR, this might tailor the population of candidates to neoadjuvant chemotherapy in colon cancer. And I think the caution with MR is really that it is so technically variable, and that access is so variable at least across the United States. Variability in MR quality is a downside which we see all the time in our practice.

AM

I think the other downside is that MR is probably harder in the abdomen when considering more mobile structures when compared to the rectum, where structures are more static. In the peritoneal disease population, MR can be harder at times to interpret because of how mobile the small bowel is, even with the use of glucose. My statement was just about the not small risk of overtreatment based on CT alone in determining the extent of the disease.

LS

I agree on this, and the other comment I wanted to make is that the advantages associated with neoadjuvant treatment might depend exactly on overtreatment, as if sort of repeating the German trial, where you could argue that some of the oncologic advantages associated with neoadjuvant treatment could depend on overtreatment, for example, treating a patient that was actually stage I rectal cancer instead of stage II or stage III.

Surgery for Locally Recurrent Colon Cancer

23

Swartjes H, van Lankveld DWP, van Erning FN, Verheul HMW, de Wilt JHW, Koëter T, Vissers PAJ. Locoregionally recurrent colon cancer: how far have we come? A population-based, retrospective cohort study. Ann Surg Oncol. 2023;30(3):1726–34.

Abstract

Background: The reported outcomes of locoregionally recurrent colon cancer (LRCC) are poor, but the literature about LRCC is scarce and aged. Recent population-based studies to provide current insight into LRCC are warranted. This study aimed to provide an overview of the incidence, risk factors, treatment, and overall survival (OS) of patients with LRCC after curative resection of stage I–III primary colon cancer.

Methods: Data on disease recurrence were collected for all patients with a diagnosis of non-metastasized primary colon cancer in the Netherlands during the first 6 months of 2015. Patients who underwent surgical resection (*N* = 3544) were included in this study. The 3-year cumulative incidence, risk factors, treatment, and OS for patients with LRCC were determined.

Results: The 3-year cumulative incidence of LRCC was 3.8%. Synchronous distant metastases (LRCC-M1) were diagnosed in 62.7% of the patients. The risk factors for LRCC were age of 70 years or older, pT4, pN1-2, and R1-2. Adjuvant chemotherapy was associated with a decreased risk of LRCC for high-risk stage

© The Author(s), under exclusive license to Springer Nature Switzerland AG 2025
D. Colibaseanu et al., *Essential Articles in Colorectal Surgery*,
https://doi.org/10.1007/978-3-031-77745-5_23

II and stage III patients [hazard ratio (HR), 0.47; 95% confidence interval (CI) 0.31–0.93]. The median OS for the patients with LRCC was 13.1 months (95% CI 9.1–18.3 months). Curative-intent treatment was given to 22.4% of the LRCC patients, and the subsequent 3 years OS was 71% (95% CI 58–87%). The patients treated with palliative treatment and best supportive care showed 3-year OS rates of 15% (95% CI 7.0–31%) and 3.7% (95% CI 1.0–14%), respectively.

Conclusions: The cumulative incidence of LRCC was low, and adjuvant chemotherapy was associated with a decreased risk for LRCC among targeted patients. Curative-intent treatment was given to nearly 1 in 4 LRCC patients, and the OS for this group was high.

DC

As with most population-based studies, this study comes from the Netherlands. As of this writing, it is the most recent study and probably one of the best written. The overarching story is the same, but some of the details are interesting and bear further discussion.

Overall, the 3554 patients here are followed for just over 3.5 years and all had stages I–III colon cancers. The patients have excellent resections with a microscopically negative margin in 97.6% of the cases. Adjuvant chemotherapy was administered to 87.7% of stage III cancers and 11.7% of stage II cancers. The locally recurrent (LR) rate was 3.8% at 3 years. Of those, 37.3% had isolated local recurrences, and 62.7% had synchronous distant metastases. LR was over 5 times higher in stage II disease compared to stage I and 14 times higher in stage III. One interesting fact was that contrary to other studies, the sidedness of cancer did not have an effect on the rate of recurrence [1, 2].

The risk factors for LR were older age, T4 tumors, N+, positive margins, lymphovascular invasion, and poor tumor differentiation. One staggering statistic is that of the patients that recurred, only 22% received an intention to cure surgery. Patients that recurred within one year of primary resection did the worst.

Still, the overall recurrence rate in this study was only 3.8% at 3 years which is less than half of what is usually reported in the literature [3].

The second interesting point was that less than 1/3 of the patients with a recurrence who went on to surgery received chemotherapy. It is unclear why that is, but given that the majority of the recurrences here had concurrent metastatic disease, additional chemotherapy would probably be helpful, a practice more alike to the US and Canada. In the study, chemotherapy is inversely associated with the risk of a LR. This strengthens the point that chemotherapy should be employed prior to resection in cases of LR.

Though it was impossible to record in this study, the location of recurrence bears some importance to the success of subsequent treatment. Anastomotic recurrences tend to be most favorable with respect to the success of resection and overall survival, while abdominal recurrences were the least favorable [4]. It may be useful to especially consider initiation of systemic therapy in cases where the recurrence is least favorable, as would be an abdominal (non-anastomotic) recurrence within one year of primary resection of a high-risk tumor (positive neurovascular invasion).

In conclusion, LR colon cancer is not well studied, and there is no uniform protocol on how to approach it. This study underscores that few of the recurrences are truly localized diseases, and even in those cases, serious consideration should be given to initiating systemic chemotherapy as the first step in approaching treating this disease.

References

1. Yang CY, Yen MH, Kiu KT, et al. Outcomes of right-sided and left-sided colon cancer after curative resection. Sci Rep. 2022;12:11323.
2. Sjövall A, Granath F, Cedermark B, Glimelius B, Holm T. Loco-regional recurrence from colon cancer: a population-based study. Ann Surg Oncol. 2007;14:432–40.
3. Storli PE, Dille-Amdam RG, Skjærseth GH, Gran MV, Myklebust TÅ, Grønbech JE, Bringeland EA. Cumulative

incidence of first recurrence after curative treatment of stage I–III colorectal cancer. Competing risk analyses of temporal and anatomic patterns. Acta Oncol. 2023;62(12):1822–30.

4. Jarrar A, Sheth R, Tiernan J, Sebikali-Potts A, Liska D, Vitello D, Kalady M, Delaney CP, Valente M, Steele SR. Curative intent resection for loco-regionally recurrent colon cancer: Cleveland clinic experience. Am J Surg. 2020;219(3):419–23.

Discussion

LS

It is impressive to see an 87.7% adherence to postoperative che-motherapy in a national population in a Western nation having a presumably high proportion of elderly individuals, even considering the relatively small size of the Netherlands. Non-adherence rates of 30% or above have been reported in large studies in the US, and the data specific for disadvantaged subpopulations and the elderly are even more sobering. I think the fragmentation of the healthcare system in the US renders implementation of guidelines on a population basis more difficult. Considering the high use of adjuvant chemotherapy following the index operations, I view these recurrences as the expression of an inherently more aggressive cancer rather than the result of a suboptimal surgical technique.

The other aspect that is a sort of the elephant in the room to me is the overall low rate of local recurrence after colon cancer. There were no comments on the surgical techniques used which I imagine were variable among the many participating hospitals. This reminds me of the controversy associated with complete meso-colic excision and whether a wide implementation of this technique would result in substantially improved outcomes. These population-based data look quite different from the dismal onco-logic outcomes of rectal cancer surgery before the widespread implementation of total mesorectal excision. The article obviously does not focus on this, but for me, as a reader, it is impossible not to think about it.

A practical aspect of this work which connects with recent data is that pT4 and incomplete resection margins after index surgery were identified as independent risk factors for local recurrence. Given the encouraging results of the FOxTROT trial if preoperative imaging suggested an elevated risk of positive resection margin and/or multivisceral resection, I would favor neoadjuvant chemotherapy. This could increase the possibility of an R0 resection which in turn could help reduce the risk of local recurrence.

MD

The data says it should be done, but the data is not definitive. Although this is obviously not a frequent occurrence, I am impressed by the absence of a clear pathway to treat these cases. I am surprised at the low rate of chemotherapy to treat locally recurrent colon cancer which is something that I would anticipate would be the expected initial approach in our practice. The other aspect that struck me is that there was no difference between right and left colon cancer. I would have imagined more variability in the management of left colon cancer than right.

AM

As has been proven again... Biology is King. I think this study highlights that from a number of factors that have already been discussed, those that have early recurrences and non-anastomotic recurrences do worse. I agree with the other sentiments that have been expressed and do feel that neoadjuvant chemotherapy in the setting of a recurrence can only benefit the patient—not just from the completeness of resection perspective, but it also allows us to test the biology of the tumor and to better understand the impact of the chemotherapeutic regimen on an overall multimodal treatment strategy. We operate far too frequently on recurrences that are truly resectable, and I think that at least in the United States, this is probably largely a function of the patients not being evaluated as completely as they should be and seeing surgeons who can truly make that decision. And I think that we see that in our own practice when probably 50% or more of patients who come here with some element of recurrence are in fact resectable when they have been told they are otherwise not resectable. And then I think, other adjuncts such as advanced metastasectomy or ablation or even now, liver transplant, increase the patient population, I think, becoming eligible for resection in the setting of recurrent disease.

LS

While I recognize the potential role of intraoperative radiotherapy in the appropriate setting, one aspect which I am not sure about is the role of HIPEC (hyperthermic intraperitoneal chemotherapy) for locally recurrent colon cancer. I am happy we work in an institution with HIPEC capabilities where we can openly discuss with our surgical oncology colleagues its possible application and plan a combined procedure as needed. I do not have a sort of ideological view of HIPEC indications in this patient population, which admittedly remains rare.

AM

There is now more emerging data on the use of HIPEC in those who have just a T4 primary colon cancer at the time of index surgery in an effort to reduce the potential likelihood of recurrence. Some of that data is relatively new so there is an element of the unknown there. In terms of radiation therapy, I mean, to me, I see a limited role in the abdomen just because more often than not, I think you can just take the local recurrence out. There are very few areas, I would imagine the vertebral bodies, which you cannot just cut out, whereas, in the pelvis, you are limited by its own bony confines. I do not think there's definitive data. Just going back to HIPEC, I do not think there's definitive data for these cases either. I mean, PRODIGE 7, which assessed primary HIPEC, had its own problems and generated a lot of criticisms. And that did change the landscape of HIPEC at least in the setting of primary disease, and perhaps, the pendulum swung too far because of the weaknesses of that trial, which inevitably would have then impacted the use of HIPEC in the locally recurrent population.

LS

In abstract terms, I am struggling with the concept of considering the peritoneum as a separate organ to be proactively addressed or does it constitute overtreatment? For example, how often would we consider prophylactic locoregional treatment of the liver without liver metastases?

AM

I guess I would say the cases I have done involved the peritoneum, so not just any locally recurrent colon cancer. If there is the involvement of the peritoneum, then I would seek out the surgical oncology colleagues' insight and consider HIPEC, and definitely, we have done that.

MD

You see these patients with multiple recurrent metastases within the abdomen.

AM

Yes, we have treated cases not limited to loco-regional recurrence of colon cancer, but also involving multiple metastases, and we have cytoreduced them, resected those metastases, and then delivered HIPEC. Admittedly there is not a lot of great data for that but adding the HIPEC probably imparts minimal additional morbidity compared to what the resection itself does.

Avoiding Surgery in Asymptomatic Patients with Stage IV Colon Cancer

24

Poultsides GA, Servais EL, Saltz LB, Patil S, Kemeny NE, Guillem JG, Weiser M, Temple LK, Wong WD, Paty PB. Outcome of primary tumor in patients with synchronous stage IV colorectal cancer receiving combination chemotherapy without surgery as initial treatment. J Clin Oncol. 2009;27:3379–84.

Abstract

Purpose: The purpose of this study was to describe the frequency of interventions necessary to palliate the intact primary tumor in patients who present with synchronous, stage IV colorectal cancer (CRC) and who receive up-front modern combination chemotherapy without prophylactic surgery.

Patients and Methods: By using a prospective institutional database, we identified 233 consecutive patients from 2000 through 2006 with synchronous metastatic CRC and an unresected primary tumor who received oxaliplatin- or irinotecan-based, triple-drug chemotherapy (infusional fluorouracil, leucovorin, and oxaliplatin; bolus fluorouracil, leucovorin, and irinotecan; or fluorouracil, leucovorin, and irinotecan) with or without bevacizumab as their initial treatment. The incidence of subsequent use of surgery, radiotherapy, and/or endoluminal stenting to manage primary tumor complications was recorded.

Results: Of 233 patients, 217 (93%) never required surgical palliation of their primary tumor. Sixteen patients (7%) required

© The Author(s), under exclusive license to Springer Nature Switzerland AG 2025

D. Colibaseanu et al., *Essential Articles in Colorectal Surgery*,
https://doi.org/10.1007/978-3-031-77745-5_24

emergent surgery for primary tumor obstruction or perforation, 10 patients (4%) required nonoperative intervention (i.e., stent or radiotherapy), and 213 (89%) never required any direct symptomatic management for their intact primary tumor. Of those 213 patients, 47 patients (20%) ultimately underwent elective colon resection at the time of metastasectomy, and eight patients (3%) underwent this resection during laparotomy for hepatic artery infusion pump placement. Use of bevacizumab, location of the primary tumor in the rectum, and metastatic disease burden were not associated with increased intervention rate.

Conclusion: Most patients with synchronous, stage IV CRC who receive up-front modern combination chemotherapy never require palliative surgery for their intact primary tumor. These data support the use of chemotherapy, without routine prophylactic resection, as the appropriate standard practice for patients with neither obstructed nor hemorrhaging primary colorectal tumors in the setting of metastatic disease.

LS

This is the fundamental study which consolidated the role of initial chemotherapy for stage IV colorectal cancer patients instead of surgery. This has been a widely debated topic for a long time, and the traditional teaching was that it was oftentimes necessary to resect the primary disease even when the patient was poorly symptomatic or asymptomatic because of the risk of subsequent obstruction, perforation, or bleeding. The other putative rationale for resection of the primary tumor would be tumor debulking to allow prolonged survival. Although in a retrospective fashion over the span of 7 years, the authors indicated that out of 233 consecutive patients with synchronous metastatic colorectal cancer and unresected primary tumor, 93% never required emergent surgery. The remaining 7% required emergent surgery for primary tumor obstruction or perforation. This is a particularly difficult group of patients to study given that in retrospective studies, patients undergoing palliative surgery tend to be fitter than patients receiving initial chemotherapy. Stage IV disease group is a heterogeneous group including for example patients with widely metastatic disease who could not tolerate either surgery or chemotherapy and are unfortunately toward the end of their lives but also patients who experience substantial tumor response after upfront chemotherapy and ultimately undergo surgery with curative intent which was actually the case for 20% of patients in this study. Most patients probably fall in between these two subgroups. The other significant variable in this debate has been the evolution of available agents for chemotherapy beyond fluoropyrimidines which has offered more effective treatment options to clinicians. Subsequent data from randomized clinical trials have corroborated the approach proposed in this article. The Japanese JCOG 1007 trial randomized 165 patients and indicated no survival benefits associated with primary tumor resection. Patient accrual was discontinued because of futility after a median follow-up of 22 months based on the recommendation of the Data and Safety Monitoring Committee [1]. The European CAIRO4 trial showed increased 60-day mortality among patients who underwent primary tumor resection followed by chemotherapy when compared with patients receiving upfront chemotherapy without surgery [2]. The more recent SYNCHRONOUS trial also confirmed the lack of benefits associated with primary tumor resection after randomization of 393 patients treated in 100 different centers and followed for a median follow-up of 36.7 months [3].

References

1. Kanemitsu Y, Shitara K, Mizusawa J, Hamaguchi T, Shida D, Komori K, Ikeda S, Ojima H, Ike H, Shiomi A, Watanabe J, Takii Y, Yamaguchi T, Katsumata K, Ito M, Okuda J, Hyakudomi R, Shimada Y, Katayama H, Fukuda H; JCOG Colorectal Cancer Study Group. Primary tumor resection plus chemotherapy versus chemotherapy alone for colorectal cancer patients with asymptomatic, synchronous unresectable metastases (JCOG1007; iPACS): a randomized clinical trial. J Clin Oncol. 2021;39(10):1098–1107.

2. van der Kruijssen DEW, Elias SG, Vink GR, van Rooijen KL, 't Lam-Boer J, Mol L, Punt CJA, de Wilt JHW, Koopman M; CAIRO4 Working Group. Sixty-day mortality of patients with metastatic colorectal cancer randomized to systemic treatment vs primary tumor resection followed by systemic treatment: the CAIRO4 phase 3 randomized clinical trial. JAMA Surg. 2021;156(12):1093–1101.
3. Rahbari NN, Biondo S, Feißt M, Bruckner T, Rossion I, Luntz S, Bork U, Büchler MW, Folprecht G, Kieser M, et al. Randomized clinical trial on resection of the primary tumor versus no resection prior to systemic therapy in patients with colon cancer and synchronous unresectable metastases. J Clin Oncol. 2022;40(17_suppl). LBA3507.

Discussion

DC

This was a great paper—even though it has been more than 14 years since it was published, it is still valid today. It really makes the point that the focus of treatment in metastatic colorectal cancer should be the metastatic disease as opposed to the primary site with the exception of complications (bleeding or obstruction). Distal rectal cancer deserves its own discussion, and others have addressed this, and in cases of impending obstruction…radiation tends to help, and endoluminal stents are hard to deploy in distal rectal cancer- and the patients tend to tolerate those poorly. This paper is making a more general point which is very valid and applicable.

MD

I found this study remarkably impactful. It offers solid evidence for managing this patient population, allowing us to avoid surgery for the majority of patients. This spares them from the potential need for a stoma and perioperative morbidity that can be associated with the operation, which is particularly crucial for these patients whose primary treatment will be chemotherapy and for those patients who may have a very limited life expectancy and time with family and loved ones.

Moreover, it reflects the advancement of chemotherapy approaches in the last few decades. Previously, resection may have been the primary option, especially when chemotherapy was less effective, relying on single agents like 5-fluorouracil (5-FU). However, with the advent of more potent chemotherapy regimens incorporating agents like oxaliplatin and vascular endothelial growth factor (VEGF) inhibitors, medical management has become increasingly effective. This study acknowledges this progress, demonstrating that with improved therapy, many patients can be managed medically, avoiding the morbidity of surgery. Of course, there are still cases where surgery is necessary, particularly in patients experiencing bleeding or obstruction. However, for asymptomatic patients or even patients with near obstruction on imaging or endoscopy without symptoms, chemotherapy is a valid first approach.

LS

What I find interesting is that this was a single institution study, which luckily ended up changing our practice even before prospective studies were available, and subsequent prospective studies have supported its results. When this study came out, I think that there was some debate which continued for some years. As somebody who has operated on patients with metastatic disease, I can attest that it is a different population. For example, there was a previous paper from Sloan Kettering indicating that when doing a restorative right colectomy for metastatic disease, the risk of anastomotic leak was much higher than what we would expect after the same operation done with curative intent. When this article was published, referrals for palliative resections in patients with stage IV disease became less common. I think that at least in my practice, it was largely because of the culture instilled by the oncology team that we ultimately evolved in our own culture as surgeons. The oncologists are the ones who stopped referring patients with asymptomatic disease and also stopped referring patients who could have minimal symptoms, for example, minimal bleeding. Therefore, it went beyond the asymptomatic patients described in this article, and we could sense that the oncologists were more comfortable in starting chemotherapy and were much less concerned that a complication would occur during chemotherapy which could have been prevented by palliative surgery. And still, sometimes, we have to intervene during chemotherapy, but rarely so. For a large proportion of patients with stage IV disease, chemotherapy first is very appropriate and helpful to at least decrease the burden of many postoperative complications after surgery with palliative intent.

DC

A side point this article makes is regarding Avastin. This has been something that I have been interested in because it seemed to be a point of contention at times or at least it was not always clear for me. As recently as 2019, the published gastroenterology (GI) literature suggests that treatment with Avastin should not be an automatic exclusion in placing endoluminal stents. So, all of that is to say that I do not have a strong opinion against the use of Avastin if an oncologist desires to use it.

MD

Yes, I agree with you. Another point highlighted in the article regarding Avastin is that perforations associated with its use typically occur in areas of the bowel other than the primary tumor site. Therefore, prophylactic resection of the primary tumor to mitigate the risk of perforation with Avastin is not beneficial. I typically defer the decision regarding Avastin to the oncologist. The only scenario where I actively discuss its use with oncology is for patients who appear likely to undergo resection in the future. In such cases, I tend to avoid Avastin to minimize concerns about this complication during the perioperative period. Generally, whether Avastin is used or not does not influence my decision regarding the necessity of an upfront operation.

High Risk of Local Recurrence Following Local Excision of T2 Rectal Cancer

25

Rothenberger DA, Garcia-Aguilar J. Role of local excision in the treatment of rectal cancer. Semin Surg Oncol. 2000;19(4):367–75.

Abstract

Local excision (LE) of properly selected rectal cancers can provide long-term survival, with minimal morbidity, negligible mortality, and excellent functional results. The role of LE has evolved over the past century. Initially, to avoid the excessive mortality of abdominal surgery, aggressive LE was performed to control the symptoms of rectal cancer. As abdominal surgery became safer, LE was restricted for use in palliation or high-risk patients. Better preoperative tumor staging resulted in an expanded role for LE, including curative-intent treatment of selected T1-2 rectal cancers. Techniques for LE include snare polypectomy, transanal excision, transanal endoscopic microsurgery, and posterior approaches. The high local recurrence rate and compromised survival reported in modern series, despite efforts to properly select patients with cancers suitable for LE, have convinced the authors to restrict the use of curative-intent LE in good-risk patients only to the most favorable rectal cancers. Close follow-up after LE is critical, because radical surgical salvage is usually possible if recurrence is identified promptly. Whether adjuvant chemoradiation can expand the role of curative-intent LE remains controversial.

© The Author(s), under exclusive license to Springer Nature Switzerland AG 2025
D. Colibaseanu et al., *Essential Articles in Colorectal Surgery*,
https://doi.org/10.1007/978-3-031-77745-5_25

DC

Local excision (LE) for rectal cancer was a controversial topic 20 years ago, and it remains no less so now. The paper published in Seminars in Surgical Oncology by Drs. Rothenberger and Garcia-Aquilar alongside illustrates the difficulty in selecting those tumors that are appropriate for a transanal approach. They right-fully identified that predicting the exact stage of rectal cancer is difficult. They did a very careful inventory of the current data and had an easy-to-follow, logical synopsis. Leaving margin-positive tumors aside, the first question is whether we can detect those patients who are likely to have positive lymph nodes, because there is no question that they should NOT have LE. Though Magnetic Resonance Imaging (MRI) is better now, just like 20 years ago, we cannot be absolutely sure that any one specific mesorectal lymph node is truly "negative." Much was discussed about adjunctive, predictive primary mass characteristics that could put some T1 cancers into the "high risk category," and cer-tainly, Nivatvong's [1, 2] and Kikuchi's [3] contributions were very helpful here. I think their conclusion was very appropriate: "At present, curative-intent LE in good-risk patients is probably best restricted to those few, highly selected, favorable early T1 rectal cancers." We did not have sufficient information to say any-thing more than that at the time this was written, so I think this was an excellent synthesis of the available data at that time. They had their own institutional study published in the same year, fol-lowing 82 patients who had undergone LE and noted that the sur-vival rate for the T1 patients was 98%, while it was 89% for the T2 tumors, and the recurrence of the T1 tumors was 18% and double that for T2 tumors. They showed that the argument of using LE as a curative treatment for T2 tumors is a very weak argument to make [4].

This question of LE for T2 tumors remains one that has been doggedly pursued by multiple groups, and we will stay with one of the two authors for this, and in 2023, we see that ACOSOG z6041 trial results were published; here it is suggested that maybe there are circumstances in which LE can be offered to some T2 patients. Here, 79 patients had chemoradiotherapy and LE. The control was another study for T2 patients who had formal proctectomy [5]. So already we see that it is not even reasonable to perform a trial in which one of the arms is LE alone for T2 patients. At the very least, it is LE and something else; in this case, it is 54 Gy of radiation concurrent with capecitabine and oxaliplatin. The patients were carefully selected for "low risk" features which I think was prudent.

There were two outcomes of this study that were particularly interesting to me, and both of them were surprising. One, the oncological outcomes were the same—essentially—as the TME Dutch study [6], which was the surrogate control study. They have 10 years of f/u results, so I think the data is as good as it is going to get as far as follow-up. The second outcome, also a surprise, was that the Dutch study had better quality-of-life scores than the LE study despite that some of the TME patients had to have permanent colostomies. There is a thoughtful discussion as to why that might be, in part having to do with radiation sequelae, but the question that is unanswerable is if the disposition of the patients from the two different countries might be different to begin with, culturally speaking.

And so, we do have different options for T2 tumors, and from an oncologic perspective, one could consider LE resection, but the question that remains…would I offer that to my patients?

References

1. Nivatvongs S, Rojanasakul A, Reiman HM, et al. The risk of lymph node metastasis in colorectal polyps with invasive adenocarcinoma. Dis Colon Rectum. 1991;34:323–8.
2. Nivatvongs S. The malignant polyp: when is enough enough? The William C. Bernstein, M.D., Memorial Lecture. Colon and rectal surgery: principles and practice 2000: 2000 Sept. 8; Minneapolis, MN.
3. Kikuchi R, Takano M, Takagi K, et al. Management of early invasive colorectal cancer. Risk of recurrence and clinical guidelines. Dis Colon Rectum. 1995;38:1286–95.

4. Garcia-Aguilar J, Mellgren A, Sirivongs P, Buie D, Madoff R, Rothenberger D. Local excision of rectal cancer without adjuvant therapy: a word of caution. Ann Surg. 2000;231:345–51.
5. Lynn PB, Van der Valk MJM, Claassen YHM, et al. Chemoradiation and local excision versus total mesorectal excision for T2N0 rectal cancer: comparison of short-term and long-term outcomes from 2 prospective studies. Ann Surg. 2023;277:96–102.
6. Kapiteijn E, Marijnen CA, Nagtegaal ID, et al. Preoperative radiotherapy combined with total mesorectal excision for resectable rectal cancer. N Engl J Med. 2001;345:638–46.

Discussion

MD

In my opinion, given the high recurrence rates post-local excision alone, it is not a viable option for patients. Recent studies confirm this concern. Regarding whether we determine it as T1 or T2, performing a transanal excision initially allows us to assess and then decide the appropriate management. Even if it confirms T2 with low-risk features, recurrence rates of up to 30% necessitate further therapy. I favor total mesorectal excision (TME), if the patient declines chemoradiation following local excision in confirmed T2 rectal cancer cases. Despite chemoradiation potentially leading to worse functional outcomes, if patients decline TME, the data supports this approach, and I would maintain this management strategy.

LS

I think the other issue that relates to this is when pursuing TNT and organ preservation, is whether we could treat with chemoradiotherapy a T2N0 lesion, which obviously leads to the possibility of overtreating a T1 lesion if misdiagnosed as a T2 lesion. If you have an MR image that really shows the rectal wall layers and the lesion involves the muscularis layer, but it does not go beyond that, in my opinion, chemoradiotherapy and chemotherapy make sense. If you have a tumor which is 3 cm or smaller, you could do a local excision and assess the staging as you pointed out, but if it is a tumor bigger than 3 cm, especially in the low rectum, the alternative may become an abdominoperineal resection. With the OPRA trial indicating a 50% organ preservation rate after TNT in locally advanced disease, I think it is difficult to contend with this, although there is no strong data and especially no guidelines to support this approach.

AM

The fundamental crux of the problem is accurately determining the pretreatment stage. Despite widely accepted practices to pursue endorectal ultrasound for MR indeterminate early lesions, we still have situations of over- or under-staging. This is where I think the surgeon's examination, particularly digital examination, is critical. It is imperative to develop the experienced digital examination and describe the tumor—is it fixed? Is it mobile? In those circumstances where imaging is uncertain, the exam can provide additional information to guide practice.

MD

I just have significant reservations about relying solely on endorectal ultrasound for distinguishing between T1 and T2 staging. In my experience, it is rare to definitively classify a lesion as strictly T1 or T2. The accuracy limitations of MRI and endorectal ultrasound in determining T staging further complicate decision-making. These concerns underscore the challenges in confidently assessing T1 and T2 lesions with imaging.

LS

A few years ago, I had a patient with a BMI of 44 kg/m², with a preoperative diagnosis of T2N0, and the tumor was not small. It was too large for a local excision. I did an open low anterior resection, and the pathology report was T1N0 with 25 negative lymph nodes. And I had done a low anterior resection with an anastomosis at four or five cm from the anal verge, and after the patient's diverting loop ileostomy was taken down, the patient developed anterior resection syndrome, and I wonder if I could have done something different. Could this be a person adequately treated with chemoradiotherapy and chemotherapy based on cT2N0 staging? This would have been overtreatment, but I do believe that I also overtreated the patient, let alone the technical difficulty of the operation in such a patient.

AM

Even in these circumstances where it remains unclear and radical surgery is less acceptable to the patient, I think it is appropriate to pursue transanal excision for confirmation. One can then refine their approach and discussion with the patient based on the pathologic stage.

DC

What is interesting about this study is that the control group, which was a Dutch cohort that had formal resection, noted a better quality of life compared to the American interventional arm which had chemoradiation. One could make the argument that the Dutch people are just tougher, and the ones I know are certainly that, but we are likely seeing the effects of radiotherapy on the rectum. That is something to consider, and I certainly did not consider it as seriously prior to reading this study. Oncologically, based on the results of this study, I would not be able to guarantee the patient that formal resection is superior to chemoradiation, or at least I do not know for sure, and patients (in the US at least) seem to heavily prefer avoiding radical surgery.

LS

I feel we all have patients who basically decide on their own care. I had cases where after chemoradiotherapy and chemotherapy, there was a residual lesion, and the patient wanted a local excision; although it did not fit the criteria of the Z6041 local excision trial, still I did a local excision; and I had a few patients who developed terrible anal pain after local excision in a recently radiated field. This is also described and was also reported in some of the patients in the Z6041 trial. Obviously, we are aware of the functional limitations after low anterior resection, especially with colo-anal anastomosis, and this includes anterior resection syndrome. However, the degree of disability associated with rectal pain was very hard to witness from a caregiver's perspective when I encountered it for the first time following a relatively small excision of a portion of the rectal wall. Whenever I discuss this treatment strategy, on a patient with cT2N0 who returns after neoadjuvant treatment with a residual lesion which the patient asks me to remove transanally, I am certainly very vocal about the risks of local excision. I feel local excision is not a walk in the park in this particular setting, and sometimes patients come to be evaluated having this preconceived idea that it is a simple operation, while only radical resection is complex. Having said that, though, I also have seen the data on the MSK patients treated with TNT who were compared retrospectively to TME patients with respect to functional results and quality of life. The quality of life was similar, but the functional results were better after nonoperative treatment. I was trained with this idea that sphincter preservation was key, and certainly, it is so for many patients, and perhaps, it would be for me, under similar circumstances. However, I have also seen poor functional results associated with a technically successful coloanal anastomosis, and I feel at times sphincter preservation is not the best way to serve our patients, particularly the older and less fit individuals. Also, based on that, I believe I have become more open to understanding the appeal of chemoradiotherapy and chemotherapy. I think the other indication could be for some of our patients who are morbidly obese with very low rectal tumors. This at least gives us another option in a clinical scenario where surgery may not result in the best outcomes and gives the patient time to lose weight.

Transanal Minimally Invasive Surgery (TAMIS) for Rectal Lesions

26

Atallah S, Albert M, Larach S. Transanal minimally invasive surgery: a giant leap forward. Surg Endosc. 2010;24:2200–5.

Abstract

Background: Our novel approach is a hybrid between transanal endoscopic microsurgery (TEM) and single-port laparoscopy that we have termed transanal minimally invasive surgery (TAMIS). We report the clinical application of this technique and present preliminary data that show TAMIS to be an effective tool for resection of both malignant and benign lesions of the rectum.

Methods: Over a 3-month period (May–July 2009), all patients with rectal lesions who were candidates for conventional transanal excision were offered the option to undergo TAMIS resection. Patients with biopsy-proven malignant lesions were required to undergo endorectal ultrasound preoperatively to determine tumor stage. To perform TAMIS, a single-incision laparoscopic surgery port (SILS Port, Covidien) is introduced into the anal canal by applying steady manual pressure. Once seated in position, endoscopic access to the rectal vault is gained and pneumorectum is established. With this access, ordinary laparoscopic instruments, including graspers, thermal energy devices, and needle drives, are used to perform the transanal excisions.

Results: Six patients, aged 43–85 years old (mean = 59.8), underwent TAMIS resection of rectal lesions. The average dis-

© The Author(s), under exclusive license to Springer Nature Switzerland AG 2025

179

D. Colibaseanu et al., *Essential Articles in Colorectal Surgery*, https://doi.org/10.1007/978-3-031-77745-5_26

tance from the anal verge was 9.3 cm and the mean tumor diameter confirmed by pathology measured 2.93 cm. There were no conversions from TAMIS to conventional transanal excision. While the average operating time was 86 min, four of the six TAMIS resections (67%) were completed in less than 1 h. The mean set-up time was only 1.9 min and this may be one reason that the mean operative time was considerably less than the average operative time for TEM surgery (120–140 min). In short-term follow-up, there was no morbidity or mortality observed.

Conclusions: TAMIS is a feasible alternative to TEM, providing its benefits at a fraction of the cost.

LS

TAMIS has been a meaningful innovation. Transanal endoscopic microsurgery (TEM) was proposed in the 80s but was never widely used. It required a commitment, both in capital expenditure and specialized training. I would say that the most daunting part of TEM was learning how to troubleshoot the machine. TransAnal Minimally Invasive Surgery (TAMIS) was an evolution of single-incision laparoscopic surgery applied to the anal canal. It is a technically simpler platform than TEM, which is easier to set up and use but also became a more affordable alternative to TEM for the average clinical practice. Subsequently, other transanal minimally invasive platforms with a rigid endoscope more similar to TEM have been introduced. One purported advantage of TAMIS when compared to the traditional transanal excision is a clearer exposure in the insufflated rectum, which according to TAMIS advocates leads to a more accurate excision with increased rates of free resection margins [1]. However, an even more meaningful advantage is the ability to remove lesions that are located cephalad to the reach of traditional transanal excision under direct vision. The first 6 patients undergoing TAMIS who were reported in the present study had an average distance from the anal verge of 9.3 cm, and in one case, removal of the lesion required entry into the peritoneal cavity which was successfully repaired during the procedure. I feel that at least the majority of these lesions could not have been removed through a transanal excision under direct vision, let alone the peritoneal breach repair. TAMIS can be used to excise T1 rectal cancers or other neoplasms but has also become a useful tool to approach a variety of complex clinical situations such as for example reexcision of scar tissue, incomplete endoscopic removals, and positive excisional margins, and when not allowing definitive treatment, it can be a valuable adjunct in treatment decisions. Without TAMIS and in those cases where a transanal excision under direct vision is technically impossible, the surgeons might have been left with the options of observation or anterior resection. Because of TAMIS, a number of patients can be spared an anterior resection with its inherent morbidity. This technique can be difficult to apply in the most distal lesions where the camera exposure with the CO_2-insufflated rectum can become difficult. Sometimes, a hybrid procedure might be necessary where the most distal portion of a lesion is removed under direct vision and the most proximal portion is removed using TAMIS. In addition, some surgeons prefer a longer, more rigid transanal endoscopic surgery platform to treat more proximal rectal lesions which arguably allows greater stability than the traditional TAMIS. Regardless of any specific limitations, it is inconceivable to go back from TAMIS. A number of surgeons have built on this platform to introduce a novel technique of retrograde transanal excision of the rectum (taTME) which will be discussed separately. More recently, robotic TAMIS (R-TAMIS) has been described and might become the next evolution of minimally invasive transanal surgery [2].

References

1. Han J, Noh GT, Cheong C, Cho MS, Hur H, Min BS, Lee KY, Kim NK. Transanal endoscopic operation versus conventional transanal excision for rectal tumors: case-matched study with propensity score matching. World J Surg. 2017;41(9):2387–94.
2. Liu S, Contreras N, Krezalek MA, Abd El Aziz MA, Merchea A, Kelley SR, Behm K. Robotic transanal minimally invasive surgery: a single institutional experience. Updates Surg. 2022;74(3):1011–6.

Discussion

MD

This original article describing the TAMIS technique truly revolutionized our ability to perform transanal excisions of large polyps and early rectal cancers. It provided an easily accessible and reproducible platform to enable safe and effective transanal resection of these lesions. During my training, we utilized TEM, which was not only an expensive upfront cost but also challenging to troubleshoot during the operation. In comparison, TAMIS offers a straightforward approach for introducing equipment into the rectum that can easily be taught and replicated. It also allows the use of the robotic platform to address even larger and more complex tumors.

DC

At the time this article came out, TAMIS was a new alternative to TEM which worked well, but as we pointed out, it was complex to set up. When I have used TEM I found that troubleshooting it was time-consuming and, in my case, most likely because I was not using it frequently enough. Versus TAMIS which was essentially laparoscopic surgery. TAMIS itself was not overly difficult, but the challenging aspect of the surgery was the closure of the defect. I could not bring myself not to close it, yet closing a large defect and especially if that defect were close to the anal verge, sometimes, that was a technical challenge.

LS

Some of my former colleagues used to warn against closure because 2 of them had patients who had experienced tumor recurrence developing from underneath the anorectal wall closure. They felt therefore that after the removal of a neoplasm, it is easier to detect a recurrence if you do not close the defect. This however was an idea applied to excision under direct vision. I think for lesions located more proximally, which is typically the case for TAMIS, especially when exposing a large area of mesorectum, the risk of bleeding increases, and there are some data about it; therefore, I do try to close the defect, which I do find to be difficult. And I have traditionally tried to avoid actually tying a knot. Now with barbed sutures, I think it is easier, but that is one of the areas where perhaps robotic surgery could make suturing easier. I think the difficulties that I found in TAMIS which I had not read about before I actually used TAMIS in practice were maintenance of the pneumorectum and bellowing. I have had some obese patients in lithotomy positions where maintaining the insufflation was a problem and the constant vibratory movement of the rectal wall created instability. With the patient in a prone position, this seems to have been less of an issue, but that has been just my experience. At times, I have added perianal skin purse string sutures around the anus and sometimes have temporarily sutured part of the perianal skin to the instrument to correct for gas leakage.

DC

With regards to the insufflation, it seemed that the air seal method did decrease some of the challenges that Luca mentioned but not completely. I would also add that it seems that with TEM getting to that full-thickness plane of dissection seemed to be faster, aforementioned technical challenges notwithstanding.

LS

I found that TEM was terrible to troubleshoot if it did not work. If it worked, it was okay. If you push the envelope on more proximal lesions with entry into the peritoneal cavity during minimally invasive transanal excision, I think that having a rigid platform consisting of a little longer tube can promote platform stability.

When you have that kind of situation, I found that if not TEM, then the Transanal Endoscopic Operations (TEO®) platform by Storz or equivalent is preferable to the actual TAMIS instrument. And perhaps with a robot, the whole paradigm will change, and it will be no longer a problem.

MD

There is a longer TAMIS platform as well which can help with stability for higher rectal lesions.

LS

Did you find that problem with the TEM platform?

MD

I only used TEM when I was in training as a resident. But did I find that the bellowing was less with TEM vs. TAMIS? Yes.

LS

Regardless of this TEM advantage, I find it very hard to imagine as a practice, to make a commitment to buy a TEM machine now. How much would we use it? It just seems that TAMIS, basically, is a branch of laparoscopic surgery. And now particularly with the possibility of doing it robotically, there is a single-port robotic platform. I think that it is difficult to conceive going back to TEM.

Lateral Lymph Node Metastatic Involvement in Rectal Cancer

27

Fujita S, Akasu T, Mizusawa J, Saito N, Kinugasa Y, Kanemitsu Y, Ohue M, Fujii S, Shiozawa M, Yamaguchi T, Moriya Y; Colorectal Cancer Study Group of Japan Clinical Oncology Group. Postoperative morbidity and mortality after mesorectal excision with and without lateral lymph node dissection for clinical stage II or stage III lower rectal cancer (JCOG0212): results from a multicentre, randomised controlled, non-inferiority trial. Lancet Oncol. 2012;13(6):616–21.

Abstract

Background: Mesorectal excision is the international standard surgical procedure for lower rectal cancer. However, lateral pelvic lymph node metastasis occasionally occurs in patients with clinical stage II or stage III rectal cancer, and therefore, mesorectal excision with lateral lymph node dissection is the standard procedure in Japan. We did a randomized controlled trial to confirm that the results of mesorectal excision alone are not inferior to those of mesorectal excision with lateral lymph node dissection.

Methods: This study was undertaken at 33 major hospitals in Japan. Eligibility criteria included histologically proven rectal cancer of clinical stage II or stage III, with the main lesion located in the rectum with the lower margin below the peritoneal reflection, and no lateral pelvic lymph node enlargement. After surgeons had confirmed macroscopic R0 resection by mesorectal

© The Author(s), under exclusive license to Springer Nature Switzerland AG 2025
D. Colibaseanu et al., *Essential Articles in Colorectal Surgery*,
https://doi.org/10.1007/978-3-031-77745-5_27

excision, patients were intraoperatively randomized to mesorectal excision alone or with lateral lymph node dissection. The groups were balanced by a minimization method according to clinical N staging (N0 or N1, 2), sex, and institution. Allocated procedure was not masked to investigators or patients. This study is now in the follow-up stage. The primary endpoint is relapse-free survival and will be reported after the primary analysis planned for 2015. Here, we compare operation time, blood loss, postoperative morbidity (grade 3 or 4), and hospital mortality between the two groups. Analysis was by intention-to-treat. This trial is registered with ClinicalTrials.gov, number NCT00190541.

Findings: 351 patients were randomly assigned to mesorectal excision with lateral lymph node dissection and 350 to mesorectal excision alone, between June 11, 2003, and Aug 6, 2010. One patient in the mesorectal excision alone group underwent lateral lymph node dissection but was analyzed in their assigned group. Operation time was significantly longer in the mesorectal excision with lateral lymph node dissection group (median 360 min, IQR 296–429) than in the mesorectal excision alone group (254 min, 210–307, $p < 0.0001$). Blood loss was significantly higher in the mesorectal excision with lateral lymph node dissection group (576 mL, IQR 352–900) than in the mesorectal excision alone group (337 mL, 170–566; $p < 0.0001$). Twenty-six (7%) patients in the mesorectal excision with lateral lymph node dissection group had lateral pelvic lymph node metastasis. Grade 3–4 postoperative complications occurred in 76 (22%) patients in the mesorectal excision with lateral lymph node dissection group and 56 (16%) patients in the mesorectal excision alone group. The most common grade 3 or 4 postoperative complication was anastomotic leakage (18 [6%] patients in the mesorectal excision with lateral lymph node dissection group vs. 13 [5%] in the mesorectal excision alone group; $p = 0.46$). One patient in the mesorectal excision with lateral lymph node dissection group died of anastomotic leakage followed by sepsis. Interpretation: Mesorectal excision with lateral lymph node dissection required a significantly longer operation time and resulted in significantly greater blood loss than mesorectal excision alone. The primary analysis will help to show whether or not mesorectal excision alone is noninferior to mesorectal excision with lateral lymph node dissection.

LS

This trial demonstrates the impact of lateral lymph nodes on local recurrence. It is truly relevant to any surgical practice despite the objective differences in the management of rectal cancer between Japan where the study was conducted and most Western countries. Patients with stage II or stage III were randomized to mesorectal excision alone vs. mesorectal excision with lateral lymph node dissection. None of the patients had suspicious lateral lymph nodes based on modern pretreatment MR of the pelvis. However, 7% of patients with mesorectal excision and lymph node dissection had lateral pelvic lymph node metastasis. This was to me the most important piece of information coming from this report, although the trial's main endpoint was to assess the noninferiority of mesorectal excision alone compared to mesorectal excision with lateral lymph node dissection. Lateral lymph node metastases have become the most common source of local recurrence of rectal cancer since the surgical technique was optimized through the introduction of total mesorectal excision. This study confirms the need to treat at least in some patients the lateral lymph nodes. For example, a total mesorectal excision with free circumferential resection margins in a patient who has mesorectal lymph node metastasis would not be sufficient as the sole treatment to address such 7% risk. In Western countries, we have addressed this through various combinations of (neo)adjuvant chemotherapy and radiotherapy for clinical stage II and III disease. The alternative could be a more systematic surgical removal of lateral lymph nodes which is more commonly performed in Japan than in the West. In a follow-up study, the 7-year recurrence-free survival rates were 71.1% after mesorectal excision with lateral lymph node dissection vs. 70.7% after mesorectal excision alone. The noninferiority of mesorectal excision alone compared to mesorectal excision with pelvic lymph node dissection could not be demonstrated. More importantly, a subgroup analysis showed a significantly improved recurrence-free survival among patients with clinical stage III disease who underwent mesorectal excision with lateral lymph node dissection compared with mesorectal excision alone [1]. This study was limited to patients with unremarkable lateral lymph nodes on initial MR staging. However, an even more complicated situation arises when any lateral lymph node is abnormal on pretreatment MR. The Lateral Node Study Consortium has indicated that for rectal cancer within the distal 8 cm from the anal verge, a node in the internal iliac compartment with a short axis of at least 7 mm on baseline MR and of more than 4 mm on MR following neoadjuvant treatment was associated with an increased risk of local recurrence. In addition, obturator lymph nodes with a short axis greater than 6 mm following neoadjuvant treatment were associated with increased distant metastasis rate and decreased cancer-specific survival. These subgroups are therefore more likely to benefit from lateral lymph node dissection [2]. The Japanese approach to lateral lymph nodes in rectal cancer has influenced our perception of rectal cancer as a disease. It also points to needed refinements in surgical technique among Western surgeons who are less familiar with lateral lymph node dissection for rectal cancer, which is technically different from the lymph node dissection performed for gynecologic or urologic malignancies. Lateral lymph node dissection and neoadjuvant treatment should not be viewed as mutually exclusive approaches, but rather as synergistic in the appropriate situation to achieve optimized cancer outcomes.

References

1. Tsukamoto S, Fujita S, Ota M, Mizusawa J, Shida D, Kanemitsu Y, Ito M, Shiomi A, Komori K, Ohue M, Akazai Y, Shiozawa M, Yamaguchi T, Bando H, Tsuchida A, Okamura S, Akagi Y, Takiguchi N, Saida Y, Akasu T, Moriya Y; Colorectal Cancer Study Group of Japan Clinical Oncology Group. Long-term follow-up of the randomized trial of mesorectal excision with or without lateral lymph node dissection in rectal cancer (JCOG0212). Br J Surg. 2020;107(5):586–94.
2. Schaap DP, Boogerd LSF, Konishi T, Cunningham C, Ogura A, Garcia-Aguilar J, Beets GL, Suzuki C, Toda S, Lee IK, Sammour T, Uehara K, Lee P, Tuynman JB, van de Velde CJH, Rutten HJT, Kusters M. Lateral Node Study Consortium. Rectal cancer lateral lymph nodes: multicentre study of the impact of obturator and internal iliac nodes on oncological outcomes. Br J Surg. 2021;108(2):205–13.

Discussion

DC

So, this was definitely an interesting question, something that I definitely wondered about for a long time. The unsurprising caveats are that it was done in Japan, by Japanese surgeons on Japanese patients. These surgeons have extensive experience with these types of lymph node dissection, so this is all to say that it is unclear how generalizable this is outside of the specific conditions it was carried under.

It seems that the randomization occurred intraoperatively, after the TME was R0. Then, it was randomized to lateral lymph node dissection vs. no lateral dissection. Without lateral lymph node dissection, the operative time was 4.2 h. With lymph node dissection, it was 6 h.

The interesting thing is that the primary outcome was disease-free survival, but this study did not look at that specifically. But the secondary outcomes were complications, and there was a higher rate of complications in the lateral lymph node dissection group. A 6-h surgery is a long surgery, and I anticipate it would be longer for me as I do not do this on a regular basis.

LS

The article was interesting to me because it changed my way of thinking about local recurrence after rectal cancer surgery. This was a trial where modern MR was used, and because of their practice in Japan, surgeons there have historically preferred lateral lymph node dissection over pelvic radiotherapy. It is a different problem than dealing with a pretreatment MR suggesting a suspicious lateral lymph node. And you had patients that had no MR evidence of lateral lymph node metastases undergoing lateral dissection and 7% had a positive lymph node. So, to me, after total mesorectal excision has been accepted and incorporated into practice, we should change the way we think about local recurrence. Patients with positive lymph nodes in the mesorectum have a substantial risk of lateral lymph node metastasis. So, this idea that you could remove the mesorectum with intact mesorectal fascia without treating the lateral lymph nodes is not sufficient. You need to do something else. And this feeds my skepticism on some of the implications of the Mercury trial on the reduction in radiotherapy use. This trial puts into perspective the risk of lateral lymph node metastases and the importance of radiotherapy in the adequate patient if you do not do lateral lymph node dissection. That is why I found that trial interesting. There is follow-up data indicating that the two approaches are comparable. So, from that perspective, perhaps, it is less relevant to a Western surgeon who would not do prophylactic lateral lymph node dissection anyway.

AM

There is a secondary paper to the main trial because this was the paper which looked at morbidity and mortality. The main trial was looking at, as you said, total mesorectal excision (TME) vs. TME with lateral pelvic lymphatic dissection. They excluded those patients who did not have clinically positive lateral nodes, and they defined clinically positive lymph nodes as greater than a centimeter in diameter, which is different than a more contemporary definition.

LS

Sure.

AM

So, in that original paper, their primary endpoint was recurrence-free survival. When they compared those who had lateral nodes versus those who did not, the local recurrence was higher, 13% vs. 7% for those who did not have lateral pelvic node dissection. But to me, the main thing about this trial is that this was all in the absence of chemotherapy and radiotherapy. And that is the biggest reason why it is not necessarily applicable to modern-day practice other than the fact that we must be cognizant, as you mentioned, of what you can say are invisible lateral positive nodes that are probably treated by chemoradiotherapy in Western practice. And in those who do not undergo chemoradiotherapy, we should still consider pursuing lateral lymph node dissection whether patients refuse chemoradiotherapy for those that qualify, but potentially even in those tumors that do not. But this trial only included stage II and stage III.

LS

This is the same trial that you mentioned, and yes, it was the first publication related to pathology results and morbidity and then the oncologic results, which actually were the objective of the trial came up later, and they were published in 2020.

MD

I agree with you, Amit. I just feel that this study is not really relevant to our practice in the United States because, especially in the era of TNT and watch-and-wait, I mean, everyone is getting neoadjuvant chemotherapy and radiation therapy with locally advanced rectal tumors, which otherwise would have treated a lot of these lateral lymph nodes. I think the other issue with this study is that not all these patients were proactively examined with an MRI. If you look at the methods, it says that they were staged with a Computed Tomography (CT) scan or MRI. And I imagine that there were many patients, especially now with better MRI technology that were missed on preoperative imaging if they were just getting a CT scan instead of an MRI which would have increased the detection rate of clinically positive lymph nodes adding to the 7% of occult lateral metastases in the study.

AM

There is a subsequent study out of Japan looking at lateral nodes for patients who had stage II and III tumors and a clinically positive lateral node, unlike this trial which included patients who do not have clinically positive lymph nodes. They looked at lateral node dissection, with or without neoadjuvant chemotherapy. All patients underwent lateral node dissection, and those who did not have neoadjuvant chemotherapy had worse overall survival and worse recurrence rates, including a worse local recurrence rate. They subsequently looked at the question for which we have some data, the MD Anderson data, on the resolution of clinically positive notes post therapy, but I think that data is very limited. We do not have any other robust data to tell us what to do with a patient who has a clinically positive node which becomes clinically negative post treatment. Do you still do a lateral node dissection or do you not? And then what do you define as clinically positive vs. negative? That is debated as well.

LS

I think this is an evolving field that is sort of germane to this study. This entity called the Lateral Node Study Consortium has found that also patients who have just four-millimeter lymph nodes following neoadjuvant treatment were at increased risk of recurrence if the lymph nodes were in the internal iliac compartment. This is a pretty specialistic kind of treatment discussion. I do not see frequently patients who need lateral lymph node dissection. And I know there's a debate about who should do it; certainly, I agree that the practices which accrued patients into this trial are different from ours, but I do feel that we should pay more attention than in the past to lateral lymph node metastases because now surgery for rectal cancer is largely optimized, at least for the accepted management of the mesorectum to reduce the risk of local recurrence. I think we do not have all the answers to these various questions of what to do with the clinical negative nodes, what constitutes clinically positive nodes, and if there is a difference between internal iliac versus obturator lymph nodes. I do not do a lateral lymph node dissection regularly, although I have treated locally recurrent rectal cancer with enlarged lymph nodes, but if this is a rare although necessary technique to use, then the question is also who should be doing this, if there should be only one person in a certain group that should be doing it. These are all questions that I think as time goes by will come to the fore.

AM

I think there is convincing data on a large number of patients indicating that those who have a positive lateral node should undergo a lateral pelvic dissection at the time of TME. I think the part that is unknown is whether this is still required if that node becomes clinically negative. The biggest trial that I know of, I think it was published in JCO in 2018, was a retrospective review of 1200 odd patients. It included those who had T3–T4 tumors and underwent TME. If they had a pretreatment MRI that showed a positive lateral node, defined as bigger or equal to 7 mm, which they saw in I think just under 20% of patients, those patients who did not undergo a lateral node dissection post treatment at the time of surgery did worse. But there was no review as to whether that node became clinically negative post treatment. Did all patients still need that or not? I think that is what is not clear. The current limited data we have would probably say, or at least I think the one that we see quoted the most from MD Anderson says they may not necessarily need that if that node becomes clinically negative. And at least that is my practice. I do not feel that you need to necessarily go after that clinically positive node which becomes clinically negative post treatment.

Robotic Surgery for Rectal Cancer

28

Jayne D, Pigazzi A, Marshall H, Croft J, Corrigan N, Copeland J, Quirke P, West N, Rautio T, Thomassen N, Tilney H, Gudgeon M, Bianchi PP, Edlin R, Hulme C, Brown J. Effect of robotic-assisted vs conventional laparoscopic surgery on risk of conversion to open laparotomy among patients undergoing resection for rectal cancer: the ROLARR Randomized Clinical Trial. JAMA. 2017;318(16):1569–80.

Abstract

Importance: Robotic rectal cancer surgery is gaining popularity, but limited data are available regarding safety and efficacy.

Objective: To compare robotic-assisted versus conventional laparoscopic surgery for risk of conversion to open laparotomy among patients undergoing resection for rectal cancer.

Design, Setting, and Participants: Randomized clinical trial comparing robotic-assisted versus conventional laparoscopic surgery among 471 patients with rectal adenocarcinoma suitable for curative resection conducted at 29 sites across 10 countries, including 40 surgeons. Recruitment of patients was from January 7, 2011, to September 30, 2014, follow-up was conducted at 30 days and 6 months, and final follow-up was on June 16, 2015.

Interventions: Patients were randomized to robotic-assisted ($n = 237$) or conventional ($n = 234$) laparoscopic rectal cancer resection, performed by either high (upper rectum) or low (total

© The Author(s), under exclusive license to Springer Nature Switzerland AG 2025
D. Colibaseanu et al., *Essential Articles in Colorectal Surgery*,
https://doi.org/10.1007/978-3-031-77745-5_28

rectum) anterior resection or abdominoperineal resection (rectum and perineum).

Main Outcomes and Measures: The primary outcome was conversion to open laparotomy. Secondary endpoints included intraoperative and postoperative complications, circumferential resection margin positivity (CRM+) and other pathological outcomes, quality of life (36-Item Short Form Survey and 20-item Multidimensional Fatigue Inventory), bladder and sexual dysfunction (International Prostate Symptom Score, International Index of Erectile Function, and Female Sexual Function Index), and oncological outcomes.

Results: Among 471 randomized patients (mean [SD] age, 64.9 [11.0] years; 320 [67.9%] men), 466 (98.9%) completed the study. The overall rate of conversion to open laparotomy was 10.1%. The overall CRM+ rate was 5.7%. Of the other, 8 reported prespecified secondary endpoints, including intraoperative complications, postoperative complications, plane of surgery, 30-day mortality, bladder dysfunction, and sexual dysfunction, none showed a statistically significant difference between groups.

Conclusions and Relevance: Among patients with rectal adenocarcinoma suitable for curative resection, robotic-assisted laparoscopic surgery, as compared with conventional laparoscopic surgery, did not significantly reduce the risk of conversion to open laparotomy. These findings suggest that robotic-assisted laparoscopic surgery, when performed by surgeons with varying experience with robotic surgery, does not confer an advantage in rectal cancer resection.

MD

The Robotic vs. Laparoscopic Resection for Rectal Cancer (ROLARR) trial published in 2017 was a randomized controlled trial comparing laparoscopy to robotic surgery for low rectal cancer. This remains the largest RCT comparing these two surgical techniques in rectal cancer. The primary endpoint was the rate of conversion to open surgery. The study was powered based on an anticipated 25% conversion rate following conventional laparoscopic surgery, given the 34% conversion rate of the previously mentioned CLASICC trial, the best available evidence at the time of the original ROLARR design, and accounting for advances in surgical technology. Four hundred and seventy-one patients were randomized to either robotic or laparoscopic surgery. The overall positive CRM rate was 5.7%. There was no difference in the conversion rate between the two groups [12.2 % laparoscopic vs. 8.1% robotic (unadjusted difference in proportions 4.1% [95% CI, −1.4% to 9.6%]) and no difference with respect to odds of conversion (adjusted OR = 0.61 [95% CI, 0.31–1.21] P = 0.16)]. There were no differences in any secondary outcomes including positive CRM rate, intraoperative complications, postoperative complications, 30-day mortality, bladder dysfunction, and sexual dysfunction. A subgroup analysis limited to male patients indicated a statistically significant difference in conversion rates favoring robotic surgery (robotic 8.7% vs. laparoscopic 16%, CI: 0.1–14.6). The authors concluded that robotic surgery does not confer any significant benefit over laparoscopy in rectal cancer. However, ROLARR ended up being underpowered based on its actual conversion rates. In addition, the participating surgeons might have been experts in conventional laparoscopic surgery but still in their learning curve in robotic surgery, thus confounding the study results.

The ROLARR trial was published during my chief year of general surgery residency and had a significant impact on my training as I entered fellowship. Due to the results of this study and I am sure many other factors unbeknownst to me, my program did not emphasize or invest in a robotics program. As a result, I had minimal robotic training in fellowship. I had a significant amount of robotic training during my general surgery residency, and so despite having limited exposure in fellowship, I was able to use robotics in my practice early on. Though this study did not show a benefit of robotic surgery compared to laparoscopy, it importantly did not show any difference in short-term oncologic or perioperative outcomes, and so despite the increased cost associated with robotics, I implemented robotic surgery into my practice. Due to limited availability, I used robotics primarily for the pelvis and rectal cancer. A significant factor in being able to do an appropriate laparoscopic TME, especially for a low pelvic tumor, is having a good first assistant. This is not always possible depending on the type of institution one is practicing in, which was the situation I was in when I first started practice. In addition to improved visualization and dexterity, the robotic platform allows the surgeon to perform an appropriate TME with much less assistance, thus enabling the surgeon to have the ability to perform an MIS procedure that may have not been possible with laparoscopy and an inexperienced assistant. So, although the ROLARR study did not show significant differences in outcomes between laparoscopy and robotics, it is still highly beneficial in these situations. Where it did show benefit was for those very challenging cases in male patients with a high BMI. ROLARR remains the largest randomized controlled trial evaluating robotics vs. laparoscopy in rectal cancer; however, since its publications, there have been several studies confirming equivalent oncologic outcomes between laparoscopy and robotics and furthermore showing benefits of robotic surgery including decreased conversion to open and improved functional outcomes [1–3]. With this data, I think that the robotic platform will only continue to show benefits as surgeons become more experienced with this technology and as technology in robotics continues to evolve.

References

1. Muaddi H, Hafid ME, Choi WJ, Lillie E, de Mestral C, Nathens A, et al. Clinical outcomes of robotic surgery compared to conventional surgical approaches (laparoscopic or open): a systematic overview of reviews. Ann Surg. 2021;273(3):467–73.
2. Lam J, Tam MS, Retting RL, McLemore EC. Robotic versus laparoscopic surgery for rectal cancer: a comprehensive review of oncological outcomes. Perm J. 2021;25:21.050.
3. Flynn J, Larach JT, Kong JCH, Waters PS, McCormick JJ, Warrier SK, et al. Patient-related functional outcomes after robotic-assisted rectal surgery compared with a laparoscopic approach: a systematic review and meta-analysis. Dis Colon Rectum. 2022;65(10):1191–204.

Discussion

MD

This study was published toward the end of my residency and had a significant impact on my training. Despite the initial enthusiasm surrounding robotics, particularly in reducing conversion rates, the study did not yield the expected results. Consequently, during my fellowship training, exposure to robotic procedures was limited, and the emphasis continued with laparoscopy. While there were likely other contributing factors unbeknownst to me, the perceived cost-benefit analysis appeared to be a significant consideration.

Since its publication, this study has been criticized for its underpowered analysis and differences in expertise between robotic and laparoscopic approaches. I think with advancements in robotic technology and increased surgeon experience, it is plausible that the results of such a study conducted today could differ favoring robotics. Moreover, subsequent research from single-institution studies has highlighted the potential benefits of robotics, including decreased conversion to open surgery and improved functional outcomes.

In my clinical practice, the benefits of robotic surgery are particularly pronounced in the pelvis, cases involving obese patients, and for performing intracorporeal anastomosis and suturing. The robotic platform affords me the ability to undertake minimally invasive procedures, even in the most complex scenarios, which in my hands would be nearly impossible with laparoscopy, especially in the absence of an experienced assistant. While this study may not have shown a significant benefit of robotics, the continued adoption of robotics, despite its costs, suggests that its benefits, particularly for specific patient demographics like males and the obese, are still recognized and valued.

LS

I do feel that you can see better in the pelvis in robotic surgery. In my early and still recent robotic experience, I had a patient in whom I encountered pelvic bleeding while dissecting the rectum. I decided to convert to open, and I could not believe how small the pelvis was when I converted. It was a very different experience from laparoscopic surgery, I can tell you that. Another important aspect of robotic surgery is fatigue, especially for older surgeons. I think that robotic surgery is easier on your body than laparoscopic surgery. You can end up having to position your body in a sort of twisted position to retract a certain structure or to look at the monitor. In robotic surgery, this is not the case.

MD

With regard to cost, as more robotic platforms are introduced into the market, I anticipate that this will gradually mitigate some of the initial costs associated with implementing robotic systems. I agree that cost remains a relative factor, contingent upon the institution and geographic location. In addition, Intuitive now offers alternatives to upfront purchases, allowing for contractual arrangements, almost like a rental agreement. This undoubtedly influences the overall cost considerations, particularly depending on one's workplace or training environment.

DC

From my perspective, just looking at the trial, I think that this was probably viewed with similar enthusiasm as Z 6051 (laparoscopic vs. open proctectomy trial). I think that in many ways, the horse was out of the barn, so to speak, at least for those surgeons who had adopted robotic surgery with enthusiasm. The patients also started asking about robotic surgery. Regardless whether robotic surgery can be shown to be superior or at least not inferior to laparoscopic technique, it was going to be adopted. And I would say that younger surgeons are more likely to learn the robot rather than laparoscopic, which is backwards from when I was trained. I think it is a great tool in the pelvis. It has definitely shown that over time, it has technical advantages, as well as the biomechanical advantages that you both talked about with respect to the surgeon. With regards to its use elsewhere in the abdomen, there are multiple camps and multiple opinions, but I do not think that there is any doubt that it has advantages in the pelvis anymore.

LS

I am aware that we will discuss the ACOSOG rectal cancer trial separately, and I see your point that indeed there are parallels between the ACOSOG trial and the ROLARR trial. However, for me personally, I come from a different perspective. When the ACOSOG trial started, it was supposed to confirm the advantages of laparoscopic surgery in rectal cancer, and there was this sense, an expectation that this was going to be the result, because it had been clear from multiple randomized trials in colon cancer that laparoscopic surgery was better. However, we realized that this was not the case. I know some details of the ACOSOG trial because I entered patients into it and was therefore an active participant. I think that the ACOSOG trial was more coherent than ROLARR in its organization and accrual, because the participants in part overlapped with the participants in the previous COST colon trial, of which ACOSOG was a sort of extension. And the other thing for the ACOSOG is that there was an immediate counterpart from Australia which was published essentially at the same time, and that trial showed similar results in Australasia. How can you be more scientific than this? In the ROLARR, I agree with your comments about the level of expertise among participants in laparoscopic vs. robotic surgery. In a way, I think that the ROLARR trial put the robotic arm at a disadvantage so that I view the ROLARR as confirmatory of the adequacy of robotic surgery, whereas at least for me the ACOSOG was a setback on the promises of laparoscopic surgery. Not even in the recovery parameters and hospital discharge was laparoscopic surgery better than open surgery for rectal cancer in the ACOSOG trial. So, for me, the question became why should we sweat so much and give our patients no tangible benefit?

MD

When both studies were released, my thought process was pretty similar. I distinctly recall reviewing the ACOSOG trial during a journal club session while I was a resident. Upon closer examination of the study details, it became evident that the findings leaned more toward being inconclusive rather than definitive, raising concerns about the oncologic safety of laparoscopy in rectal cancer. Conversely, the ROLARR trial essentially affirmed the safety of robotic surgery but fell short of demonstrating a clear superiority of the technique over laparoscopy, which sparked controversy over whether the investment in robotic technology was warranted. Nonetheless, there was generally less uncertainty regarding the safety and efficacy of robotic surgery compared to laparoscopy in my opinion.

Transanal Total Mesorectal Excision (taTME) for Rectal Cancer

29

Wasmuth HH, Faerden AE, Myklebust TÅ, et al. Transanal total mesorectal excision for rectal cancer has been suspended in Norway. Br J Surg. 2020;107(1):121–30.

Abstract

Background: Transanal total mesorectal excision (TaTME) for rectal cancer has emerged as an alternative to the traditional abdominal approach. However, concerns have been raised about local recurrence. The aim of this study was to evaluate local recurrence after TaTME. Secondary aims included postoperative mortality, anastomotic leak, and stoma rates.

Methods: Data on all patients who underwent TaTME were recorded and compared with those from national cohorts in the Norwegian Colorectal Cancer Registry (NCCR) and the Norwegian Registry for Gastrointestinal Surgery (NoRGast). Kaplan–Meier estimates were used to compare local recurrence.

Results: In Norway, 157 patients underwent TaTME for rectal cancer between October 2014 and October 2018. Three of seven hospitals abandoned TaTME after a total of five procedures. The local recurrence rate was 12 of 157 (7.6%); eight local recurrences were multifocal or extensive. The estimated local recurrence rate at 2.4 years was 11.6% (95% c.i. 6.6–19.9) after TaTME compared with 2.4% (1.4–4.3) in the NCCR ($P < 0.001$). The adjusted hazard ratio was 6.71 (95% c.i. 2.94–15.32). Anasto-

© The Author(s), under exclusive license to Springer Nature Switzerland AG 2025
D. Colibaseanu et al., *Essential Articles in Colorectal Surgery*,
https://doi.org/10.1007/978-3-031-77745-5_29

motic leaks resulting in reoperation occurred in 8.4% of patients in the TaTME cohort compared with 4.5% in NoRGast ($P = 0.047$). Fifty-six patients (35.7%) had a stoma at latest follow-up; 39 (24.8%) were permanent.

Conclusion: Anastomotic leak rates after TaTME were higher than national rates; local recurrence rates and growth patterns were unfavorable.

LS

This is a publication which has corroborated the apprehension of many surgeons regarding this technique. The idea of approaching the rectum from the perineum in a retrograde, minimally invasive fashion to facilitate deep pelvic dissection especially in an obese male patient makes intuitive sense, and I admire the pioneers who conceived the feasibility of this technique [1] and those who put their effort to understand its applicability. This article focuses on the oncologic outcomes following transanal total mesorectal excision (taTME), which are obviously paramount, and it is concerning to read that trained surgeons did try and apply this technique only to reach such a drastic consensus in a whole country, albeit one with a population of less than 5.5 million. To be fair, the oncologic data from the International taTME Registry based on 2803 patients operated in 203 centers worldwide indicate that this technique is associated with low rates of positive circumferential resection margin and high rate of mesorectal completeness. The two-year local recurrence rate was 4.8%, but only 4% of the local recurrence cases had a multi-site pelvic recurrence pattern [2]. I have never applied this technique for cancer, and therefore, I cannot comment on any personal surgical experience. However, I feel I can comment on the dilemma of somebody who could embark on learning a new technique with the expectation that it will serve our patients better. The taTME technique seems to be difficult to learn and is associated with specific complications such as urethral injuries and CO_2 embolism that I would feel are less common at least when learning anterior resection using other techniques. The reported anastomotic leak rate seemed at times higher than what would be expected after alternative approaches, but to its credit, the International taTME Registry has used a very liberal definition of anastomotic leak [3]. The International consensus on taTME guidelines indicates that taTME should be used in rectal cancers only when TME is indicated, and a transanal approach should be recommended in rectal cancer patients where a clear distal margin cannot be guaranteed by a pure abdominal approach [4]. However, one puzzling aspect of some publications on taTME is that there seems to be a tendency toward performing a lower anastomosis, even for relatively proximal rectal tumors, located up to 14 cm from the anal verge in the taTME Registry [3]. A critic might view this as an example of the patient fitting the operation rather than vice versa so that some patients could have safely retained a few more centimeters of rectum which could help to preserve their defecatory function. The prospective randomized TaLaR trial from China compared taTME and laparoscopic rectal among patients having rectal cancer at a mean distance of 5.2 cm from the anal verge, which was comparable between the groups. The taTME group was associated with a significantly greater proportion of handsewn colo-anal anastomoses, while laparoscopic surgery was associated with a significantly greater proportion of stapled anastomoses [5]. An issue related to indications of taTME is taTME applicability. If we consider the spectrum of rectal cancer, there are of course more proximal tumor locations and patients having poor sphincter function which are not candidates for a restorative procedure. Abdominoperineal resection using taTME technique is possible but not frequently performed [2]. Once we assume that taTME is truly applied only to lower rectal cancer, we need to consider the initial learning curve and also expect that a surgeon should do several taTME cases a year to maintain clinical expertise. Therefore, how many colorectal surgeons have a kind of practice heavily skewed toward distal rectal cancer, not to mention general surgeons who frequently operate on rectal cancer, at least in the United States? The applicability of this new technique might be limited, and the successful results of a few experts might not be sufficient to propel taTME to become the new standard of care, supplanting both the other minimally invasive options and open surgery. Further study on taTME remains necessary. Other ongoing trials such as COLOR III and GRECCAR 11 will provide additional data on the outcomes associated with this technique.

References

1. Sylla P, Rattner DW, Delgado S, Lacy AM. NOTES transanal rectal cancer resection using transanal endoscopic microsurgery and laparoscopic assistance. Surg Endosc. 2010;24(5):1205–10.
2. Roodbeen SX, Penna M, van Dieren S, Moran B, Tekkis P, Tanis PJ, Hompes R; International TaTME Registry Collaborative. Local recurrence and disease-free survival after transanal total mesorectal excision: results from the International TaTME Registry. J Natl Compr Canc Netw. 2021;19(11):1232–40.
3. Penna M, Hompes R, Arnold S, Wynn G, Austin R, Warusavitarne J, Moran B, Hanna GB, Mortensen NJ, Tekkis PP; International TaTME Registry Collaborative. Incidence and risk factors for anastomotic failure in 1594 patients treated by transanal total mesorectal excision: results from the International TaTME Registry. Ann Surg. 2019;269(4):700–11.
4. TaTME Guidance Group representing the ESCP (European Society of Coloproctology), in collaboration with the ASCRS (American Society of Colon and Rectal Surgeons), ACPGBI (Association of Coloproctology of Great Britain and Ireland), ECCO (European Crohn's and Colitis Organisation), EAES (European Association of Endoscopic Surgeons), ESSO (European Society of Surgical Oncology), CSCRS (Canadian Society of Colorectal Surgery), CNSCRS (Chinese Society of Colorectal Surgery), CSLES (Chinese Society of Laparo-Endoscopic Surgery), CSSANZ (Colorectal Surgical Society of Australia and New Zealand), JSES (Japanese Society of Endoscopic Surgery), SACP (Argentinian Society of Coloproctology), SAGES (Society of American Gastrointestinal and Endoscopic Surgeons), SBCP (Brazilian Society of Coloproctology), Swiss-MIS (Swiss Association

for Minimally Invasive Surgery). International expert consensus guidance on indications, implementation and quality measures for transanal total mesorectal excision. Colorectal Dis. 2020;22(7):749–55.

5. Liu H, Zeng Z, Zhang H, Wu M, Ma D, Wang Q, Xie M, Xu Q, Ouyang J, Xiao Y, Song Y, Feng B, Xu Q, Wang Y, Zhang Y, Hao Y, Luo S, Zhang X, Yang Z, Peng J, Wu X, Ren D, Huang M, Lan P, Tong W, Ren M, Wang J, Kang L; Chinese Transanal Endoscopic Surgery Collaborative (CTESC) Group. Morbidity, mortality, and pathologic outcomes of transanal versus laparoscopic total mesorectal excision for rectal cancer short-term outcomes from a multicenter randomized controlled trial. Ann Surg. 2023;277(1):1–6.

Discussion

DC

I have to say that when this came out, I was pretty excited about it. I was already using the robot, but maybe at the time, its role in rectal cancer surgery had not taken off to where it is now, and I was less experienced with the robot. So, I thought the answer for the distal rectal tumors had come, and I got certified, and I was trained. I did the course, and then I did a few cases, and fortunately, no complications. However, when I was doing the cases, I realized anteriorly is kind of tricky, and then later, it came out that there were urethral injuries, and I realized it was not just my impression that the anterior plane was tricky. In fact, it was the impression of many others. And then the robot took off and I realized that, lo and behold, getting to the pelvis is not really that big of a deal with the robot. We do it with the laparoscopic approach, too, but my neck and back definitely do not like that. I think that the robot took some of the excitement of the taTME away along with the realization there could be complications which had not been previously demonstrated, at least in the US. In addition, there was another question that still lingered. Are we starting to do, say, mid-rectal tumors with taTME, which we should not?

Because the end result of a taTME is necessarily a coloanal anastomosis, and we all know that especially with a handsewn technique, it is not the best anastomosis for function. Subsequent studies have shown that taTME is feasible, and I found myself that it can work. However, I think that training a new surgeon straight out of fellowship on taTME is not a walk in the park, and their first 20–30 cases are not going to be easy. And I found out, with the advent of the robot, I have not used taTME. I have not had the need to use it.

AM

This moratorium in Norway obviously was based upon oncologic results that they saw and on complications. I went to the course and trained in taTME, but do not use it in practice. However, I think it is a tool in the toolbox. I think when we think of rectal cancer surgery, there has always been debate upon modalities, and as training paradigms shift, modalities which were being taught shifted from open to minimally invasive. With the greater uptake in robotics compared to laparoscopic, we have seen that minimally invasive rectal cancer surgery has proportionally increased. Where do you place taTME in this? I think it is a tool that, for those who are adequately trained and practice it in a high volume manner, is not associated with the complication rate that has been reported out of Norway, and it does potentially have a similar oncologic outcome, although the long-term results are not yet available.

After this Norway moratorium, there has been a multicenter trial led by Patricia Sylla which looked at taTME in low rectal cancers and at least found that when performed by expert taTME surgeons, it seemed to be safe. And I think my only comment in terms of functional outcomes is that I do not think we really know with robust data what the true functional outcomes are.

I am suspicious as he is in terms of functional outcome data, given the low anastomoses. But the difference between handsewn coloanal anastomosis and taTME is that with taTME, unless you are doing an intersphincteric resection, you are preserving the anal transition zone in most cases. And so, by preserving that zone (that is eliminated when we are doing typical handsewn coloanal anastomosis), the function may be improved. I agree with others that with mid-rectal tumors and higher rectal tumors, this is probably not the best modality from a functional perspective. I just do not think we have enough data, at least long-term data, in low cancers to know definitive functional outcomes.

LS

I noticed that you did not mention oncologic outcomes in your concerns regarding taTME.

DC

I do not think it is inferior with respect to that, from what I have seen. With respect to Amit's comments about the urethral injuries, I wanted to say that they were actually complications found at high-volume centers, and that could have been at the beginning of their learning curve. And so, it is tough for me, when I did not do a lot of them, and though probably the most in our group, still not enough to continue doing taTME. I agree that it could be a great tool for somebody who does a lot of taTME, and it would be a great skill for somebody who specifically does a lot of low rectal cancers. I recognize that it is innovative for sure, but I do not think it would apply to my practice.

AM

There is one thing I would echo with Dorin's comments—in terms of rectal cancer surgery that goes beyond taTME. I think whichever modality any surgeon chooses, they really have to be doing it in sufficient volume to be competent, whether that's open, laparoscopic, robotic, or transanal technique.

DC

Absolutely, you are 100% correct.

MD

I think the issue with taTME is that the idea of using it to approach the low pelvis is good. But I think this study, which shows this concern about increased local recurrence compared to other studies that have not shown this, really speaks to the fact that this is a very technically demanding procedure which is not easily replicated and is only really applicable or has the most value in low, distal rectal cancers. I think it is hard to have a practice where that is all you are doing, unless you are in a country where all the rectal cancer cases are funneled to one institution, like they might have in Europe. So, when I was in training, this was just coming out. I was part of a lot of procedures carried out by surgeons who were doing it for the first time, and it is really not an easy procedure. And when I finished, I was considering whether I should do the course, and this paper came out and really supplanted my desire to put this into my practice right away. And I would echo Dorin's thoughts with regard to robotics. I think that robotics has really helped with low rectal dissection where I do not find that taTME would be of as much benefit, given the risks that are associated with it.

AM

I guess the other question that I do not think has been sufficiently answered in any research on taTME is whether it really reduces the abdomino-perineal resection (APR) rate? Robotic approaches are probably the best comparison here. Do patients who are getting taTME have a lower rate of APR?

As a surgeon who does not do taTME, I am obviously biased, but maybe one of the factors that's touted with taTME is that you have a more precise distal transection line so that you can better tailor the appropriate margin below the tumor. Does this decrease APR rates? I don't think so.

DC

I think with the robot we have an easier time with lower dissections than laparoscopically, at least for me. With a robot, low pelvic dissections are easier technically and physically. So while I think that taTME has that little sweet spot in the very low rectal cancers, maybe the robot is able to scratch that itch, if you will.

LS

With respect to the issue of the distal margin, you can dissect the mucosa or part of the sphincter as needed and do it circumferentially with the patient in lithotomy or prone position. You can temporarily expose the anus and then close the distal edge of such dissection and then go back and do the abdominal part using a robotic technique or open or laparoscopic technique depending on your preference. So, I also do not feel that the precise determination of the distal margin is a feature unique to taTME. However, the opposite is true, where in practice among many surgeons, and I am not saying among the proponents of taTME who have done it from the beginning, there is a drag toward coloanal anastomosis when it is not oncologically necessary with the negative consequences that Amit pointed out. I think that there is the issue of experience, which also Michelle alluded to, where in order for you to have the volume and the expertise in this technique, you tend to do an anastomosis more distally than you would do using any of the other options, and in doing this, you could compromise the functional results in individuals who would end up having a higher anastomosis if using another technique.

AM

Even the use of the access platform for the operation that is left in place for an extended period of time into the anus might have a detrimental effect on function. I think the other alternative to consider in these situations is a transanal transection with single stapling which I guess you could consider as maybe somewhat of a hybrid approach. Maybe you do mobilization from above in whichever manner you want to, and you can do that mobilization all the way down, basically. But you do not transect trans abdominally, and instead, you transect through the anus and then place your purse string through the anus and perform the stapling from there. You still have to obviously do the complete TME from above. And for people who are not proponents of taTME, that does not seem to be an issue, and then, you take maybe the one benefit or one of the biggest benefits of taTME and direct visualization transanally for your transaction at the appropriate distal margin.

LS

I think the advocates of taTME support this, and they say that this issue of dragging the anastomosis to coloanal should not exist, and you should be able to do taTME with a higher single-stapled anastomosis. I have never done an anastomosis using that technique, so I should be humble in presenting this, but my understanding when discussing this with people who have done it is that doing this with a single-stapled anastomosis in the context of taTME adds to the technical difficulty of this approach, and so you have an anastomosis that could be let's say at 5 cm from the anus which is pretty high if you have to put a purse string from the anus, whereas perhaps a rectal transection with a stapler from the abdomen might be, at least in individual cases, easier. So, you might end up having incomplete doughnuts or an air leak positive test because of some technical difficulties that are specifically associated with the surgeon's choice to place the purse string from the bottom and do taTME. I find this to be an added issue to consider if one wants to pursue taTME.

AM

Those are good points, and actually, the other comment about the robot is that the tools give you an easy ability to do a handsewn purse string placement trans abdominally which would be very difficult to do laparoscopically.

The Complex Management of Enterocutaneous Fistula

30

Lynch AC, Delaney CP, Senagore AJ, Connor JT, Remzi FH, Fazio VW. Clinical outcome and factors predictive of recurrence after enterocutaneous fistula surgery. Ann Surg. 2004;240(5):825–31.

Abstract

Objective: Recent experience with surgery for enterocutaneous fistulae (ECF) at a specialist colorectal unit is reviewed to define factors relating to a successful surgical outcome.

Summary of Background Data: ECF cause significant morbidity and mortality and need experienced surgical management. Previous publications have concentrated on mortality resulting from fistulae, while factors affecting recurrence have not previously been a focus of analysis.

Methods: Records were reviewed of patients who had ECF surgery (1994–2001). Management strategy involved early drainage of sepsis and nutritional support prior to elective ECF repair, with selective defunctioning proximal stoma formation.

Results: A total of 205 patients were available (89 males, 43%; median age, 51 years; range, 16–86 years). ECF were related to Crohn's disease in 95, ulcerative colitis in 18, diverticular disease in 17, carcinoma in 25 (16 after radiotherapy), mesh ventral hernia repair in 21, and other causes in 29. Forty-one (20%) had undergone attempted fistula repair at other institutions. Initial management included CT-guided drainage of an intra-abdominal abscess in 23 patients, and total parenteral nutrition in 74 (36%). A total of

© The Author(s), under exclusive license to Springer Nature Switzerland AG 2025
D. Colibaseanu et al., *Essential Articles in Colorectal Surgery*,
https://doi.org/10.1007/978-3-031-77745-5_30

203 patients had definitive ECF repair. Forty-four had oversewing or wedge resection of the fistula, and 159 had resection and reanastomosis of the involved small bowel segment or ileocolic anastomosis. Ninety-day operative mortality was 3.5%. A total of 42 (20.5%) patients developed ECF recurrence within 3 months. Multivariate analysis demonstrated that recurrence was more likely after oversewing (36%) than resection (16%, $P = 0.006$).

Conclusions: A strategy of drainage of acute sepsis, maintenance of nutritional support prior to surgery, and selective use of PS allows primary closure in 80% of complicated ECF. Resection should be performed when feasible.

LS

This is a large study conducted by a group with considerable experience in this field. Management of ECF requires extensive preoperative care to optimize postoperative outcomes. In this series, the ECF had been present for a median of 5.8 months prior to the index procedure. This is an appropriate interval to reduce the adverse effect of intrabdominal adhesions from previous laparotomy, although some surgeons accept 3 or 4 months. All synchronous abdomino-pelvic abscesses should be drained whenever possible before any elective operations. A percutaneous drain might be left in place until the day of surgery if it controls an internal fistulous opening in addition to the ECF. Thirty-six percent of patients received total parenteral nutrition (TPN) before their elective surgery. TPN is necessary for nutritional optimization, but also to alleviate the skin damage associated with ECF, particularly in the case of high-output fistula. In these situations, TPN duration can therefore exceed the 7–10 days typically necessary to strictly optimize nutrition in anticipation of elective surgery and abdominal closure. It is notable that the largest subgroup out of 205 patients in the series consisted of 95 individuals who had enterocutaneous fistula (ECF) associated with Crohn's disease. This is unusual when compared to other series where ECF developed postoperatively in 89.4% of cases [1]. In patients with Crohn's disease, preoperative medical management including biologic medications can contribute to controlling the activity of the disease and aiding in preoperative optimization. The multivariate analysis indicated that recurrence was more likely after over-sewing the fistula defect when compared to resection of the segment containing the fistula. This is not surprising, and the authors specifically point out in the discussion that the decision to oversew rather than resect the fistula defect could have been dictated by prohibitive scarring of the peritoneal cavity which prevents lysis of adhesions at the risk of creating enterotomies and increasing intraoperative bleeding. This is a sometimes difficult decision to make intraoperatively, which depends on the individual surgeon's experience and personal approach to ECF. Of course, it would be ideal to amply dissect the segment to be resected followed by an anastomosis of 2 segments of viable, healthy bowel. The authors also discuss the use of a defunctioning ileostomy in addition to primary ECF management. Especially after multiple resections involving the more proximal small bowel and/or in case of multiple enterotomies, it may be necessary to create a diverting jejunostomy, which is not specifically mentioned in this publication. This comes inevitably associated with the need for TPN, ideally for 3 months assuming an uneventful postoperative course, after which the jejunostomy can be taken down. Even a diverting ileostomy not located in the distal small bowel can be associated with high stoma output which may be impossible to manage using only oral medications and dietary modifications, ultimately requiring TPN anyway. In those cases, my preference is to schedule the patient for a tunneled subcutaneous central line placement as soon as safe after surgery, typically on the second postoperative day. A tunneled central venous catheter, generally in a subclavian vein, is associated with a reduced risk of infection compared to a peripherally inserted central catheter (PICC), especially if TPN is prolonged beyond the ideal 3 months following ECF repair due to postoperative complications. Another controversial aspect is the use of ureteral stents. If the ECF patient had a proctectomy with a stoma, particularly in the case of total proctocolectomy and end ileostomy, it is likely that multiple small bowel loops requiring dissection are located in the pelvis, and therefore, I strongly favor ureteral stent placement. Another relevant point suggested by the study population is the management of ECF associated with previous mesh hernia repair. In this setting, a primary abdominal wall closure may be technically impossible. This is not specifically addressed in the present article but is a topic germane to ECF management. In a review examining ECF management reported in 53 studies, 315 patients underwent abdominal wall reconstruction and 72% of them required mesh [1]. The type of abdominal mesh material to be used in contaminated cases remains controversial. It is possible that biologic mesh does not provide any advantages compared to synthetic mesh [2]. One feasible option is to use Vicryl mesh to facilitate recovery after ECF repair and delay any definitive management of abdominal wall hernia. It would be ideal to approach ECF closure with much less invasive techniques such as over-the-scope closure (OTSC) [3] when technically feasible. This is a reasonable initial approach, leaving surgery as a salvage option in case of OTSC failure. Unfortunately, the majority of chronic ECF cases still require major abdominal surgery.

References

1. Gefen R, Garoufalia Z, Zhou P, Watson K, Emile SH, Wexner SD. Treatment of enterocutaneous fistula: a systematic review and meta-analysis. Tech Coloproctol. 2022;26(11):863–74.
2. Rosen MJ, Krpata DM, Petro CC, Carbonell A, Warren J, Poulose BK, Costanzo A, Tu C, Blatnik J, Prabhu AS. Biologic vs synthetic mesh for single-stage repair of contaminated ventral hernias: a randomized clinical trial. JAMA Surg. 2022;157(4):293–301.
3. Roy J, Sims K, Rider P, Grimm L, Hunter J, Richards W. Endoscopic technique for closure of enterocutaneous fistulas. Surg Endosc. 2019;33(10):3464–8.

Discussion

DC

This is a great article illustrating some of the perhaps less grandiose aspects of the colorectal surgery practice but nonetheless demonstrates that a good understanding of the relevant data and extensive experience are key. That is why these types of problems should always be treated at tertiary centers with not only the expertise but also the necessary resources to treat these difficult problems. As the authors note, resolution comes after months and in my experience sometimes years of a very meticulous and intentional approach. This requires commitment on both the part of the patient and the surgeon and team.

I would add that it is useful to think of colon fistulas and small bowel fistulas as separate identities with respect to treatment. While some of the treatments are similar (nutrition, clearing all infection, patience), the high output associated with proximal small bowel fistulas have pushed us to go to surgery sooner if adequate control is not obtained, and it is also more likely that resection is necessary. Of course, with a distal small bowel, or colonic fistulas, we always have the option of diverting proximal to any repair, which can be very useful when strategically used. However, the challenge with a colonic fistula can be managing the thickness of the output, which often time requires repeated drain exchanges to increase size, and sometimes, that is also not enough.

I find that the article is laudable in its ability to capture a somewhat heterogenous collection of fistulas and present a systematic approach in their treatment which is undoubtedly helpful to the novice colorectal surgeon as well as the experienced one.

MD

The authors looked at a wide variety of patients with different types of fistulas, whether IBD-related or radiation-induced or iatrogenic. But regardless of the ECF source, primary repair of the fistula is associated with more morbidity and recurrence of the fistula, so if at all possible, we should be trying to resect the segment with the fistula. They do acknowledge that in some situations, that is just not possible depending on the hostility of the abdomen, and so in those situations, sometimes, a primary repair is really all you can do, which I think certainly increases that risk of recurrence. I think the article goes into nice detail about everything that should be done to optimize the patient's condition prior to fistula takedown, including draining of sepsis, improving malnutrition, etc., but I think the takeaway for me was more so the surgical technique and how we can prevent recurrence of fistula after what usually is a pretty big surgery.

AM

I am a bit traumatized from residency and Dorin, I'm sure, will share some of this on the pretty entertaining patient population that the trauma critical care service in our residency program has taken care of, and I think the key factor from that which I think I learned is not really the surgery itself but the patient preparation prior to surgery. This was probably the more critical aspect of success, ranging from optimizing things like addressing undrained sepsis to healing the skin of the abdominal wall and ensuring adequate nutrition. All of that, to me, was one of the bigger factors that led to success in these patients. Probably more so than the actual takedown of the fistula.

LS

I agree, and I would also say that, at least in the cases that I have seen, there seemed to be an association which I cannot prove scientifically, but there seemed to be an association between ECF and poor socioeconomic status and/or poor access to care. Several times, these were patients who had been operated on elsewhere and had experienced ECF as a postoperative complication which they found it difficult to manage locally. This of course could be just their opinion, and there can be many factors leading to unsuccessful management of ECF. However, I do feel that it adds to the complexity and difficulty of care because it is not a population that seems to have necessarily all the support system that they would need to be given, as Michelle and Amit pointed out, the extraordinary work that is required before the actual surgery for fistula takedown can take place. I find it to be the case also within the subset of Crohn's disease patients, where oftentimes progression to perforating disease to the point of causing a disease-related ECF is also associated with lack of access to care or unrealistic confidence in the ability of medical management to control the fistula.

The Advent of Enhanced Recovery Protocols After Surgery

31

Delaney CP, Fazio VW, Senagore AJ, Robinson B, Halverson AL, Remzi FH. 'Fast track' postoperative management protocol for patients with high co-morbidity undergoing complex abdominal and pelvic colorectal surgery. Br J Surg. 2001;88(11):1533–8.

Abstract

Background: A combination of factors has emphasized the need to reduce postoperative stay after surgery. Multimodal care plans may shorten hospital stay but have been associated with high readmission rates and are generally reserved for straightforward, non-complicated colonic (not rectal) resections. This study evaluated a "fast track" protocol in patients undergoing major colonic and rectal surgery.

Methods: Sixty consecutive patients (median age 44.5 (range 13–70) years) underwent major procedures over a 6-week period on one colorectal service. Nasogastric tubes and epidural anesthesia were not used. Patients participated in a protocol of early diet and early ambulation and were discharged after meeting defined criteria.

Results: Fifty-eight patients (97%) were deemed suitable for the "fast track" approach at the time of surgery and stayed for a mean (s.d.) of 4.3 (1.6) days after operation. Patients in diagnosis-related group (DRG) 148 (colorectal resection with co-morbidity; $n = 40$) stayed for 4.6 (1.7) days, which was longer than those in

© The Author(s), under exclusive license to Springer Nature Switzerland AG 2025
D. Colibaseanu et al., *Essential Articles in Colorectal Surgery*,
https://doi.org/10.1007/978-3-031-77745-5_31

DRG 149 (without co-morbidity; $n = 18$) who stayed 3.5 (0.8) days ($P = 0.01$). Three patients (5%) required a nasogastric tube for vomiting. There were no readmissions directly attributable to "fast track" failure, although four patients (7%) were readmitted within 30 days of operation for other reasons. Eight poorly compliant patients stayed for 5.1 (1.1) days ($P = 0.02$ versus compliant patients). "Fast track" patients had a shorter length of stay than patients receiving traditional care on other colorectal services during the same time period (compared by DRG 148, DRG 149 and for all patients) ($P < 0.0001$).

Conclusion: The "fast track" protocol allows patients with high levels of co-morbidity undergoing complex colorectal and reoperative pelvic surgery to benefit from a rapid recovery and early discharge from hospital. The approach is safe and has low readmission rates.

LS

The term "fast track" precedes the more modern term of enhanced recovery protocols, but it is based on the same principles introduced in Northern Europe at the end of the 90s [1]. Enhanced recovery protocols are multimodal care plans aiming to achieve accelerated postoperative recovery, reduction of postoperative pain and therefore narcotic use, and earlier discharge from the hospital and therefore reduced hospital cost. All of this remains associated with comparable readmission rates and comparable if not decreased postoperative morbidity. This was a group of patients undergoing complex open procedures with high comorbidity rates who did not receive prophylactic nasogastric tubes postoperatively and did not receive epidural anesthesia. Pain control was based on patient-controlled analgesia, and patients were encouraged to walk and were offered oral liquids on the evening of surgery. Diet was advanced as tolerated if patients could tolerate liquids. Foley catheters were removed on postoperative day 2, and intra-abdominal suction drains were also removed unless there was a specific individual concern. Patients were discharged from the hospital once they had resumed having bowel function (flatus/gas or stool), could drink, eat solid food comfortably, and were comfortable on oral analgesia. The application of these principles resulted in shorter length of stay than among patients receiving traditional care on other colorectal services during the same period. This protocol was novel at the time of this study and was applied to their patients by experienced surgeons who were not using minimally invasive techniques and exclusively performed open colorectal operations. The results of this study speak to the effectiveness of the enhanced recovery protocol concept, although the specific interventions used have become largely obsolete during the 20 years and beyond following this publication. Multiple prehabilitation and other preoperative interventions complement today the intraoperative and postoperative protocols. The preferential use of minimally invasive techniques is recognized as quintessential to enhanced recovery protocols. Loco-regional anesthesia in some form tailored to the surgical approach (intrathecal morphine injection, transversus abdominis plane block, or thoracic epidural anesthesia for open operations) is generally recommended, while patient-controlled anesthesia has been progressively abandoned in favor of more aggressive opioid-sparing pain management plans [2]. Enhanced recovery protocols are now widely accepted. Extensive literature has confirmed its medical benefits, and the related hospital savings have been also noted in the business literature [3]. The new frontier of enhanced recovery protocols is perhaps a more widespread achievement of same-day discharge following minimally invasive colorectal surgery, which is already possible in selected patients [4].

References

1. Kehlet H, Mogensen T. Hospital stay of 2 days after open sigmoidectomy with a multimodal rehabilitation programme. Br J Surg. 1999;86(2):227–30.
2. Irani JL, Hedrick TL, Miller TE, Lee L, Steinhagen E, Shogan BD, Goldberg JE, Feingold DL, Lightner AL, Paquette IM. Clinical Practice Guidelines for Enhanced Recovery After

Colon and Rectal Surgery From the American Society of Colon and Rectal Surgeons and the Society of American Gastrointestinal and Endoscopic Surgeons. Dis Colon Rectum. 2023;66(1):15–40.

3. Larson DW. How mayo clinic got buy-in for a plan to reduce hospital stays. Harvard Business Review; 2019.

4. McLemore EC, Lee L, Hedrick TL, Rashidi L, Askenasy EP, Popowich D, Sylla P. Same day discharge following elective, minimally invasive, colorectal surgery: A review of enhanced recovery protocols and early outcomes by the SAGES Colorectal Surgical Committee with recommendations regarding patient selection, remote monitoring, and successful implementation. Surg Endosc. 2022;36(11):7898–914.

Discussion

LS

This article was important in my personal experience, because I was skeptical about the principles of what is now referred to as enhanced recovery protocols (ERPs), but I ultimately became a convert. I certainly was not a first adopter. I felt as if it was a discussion about minutiae, and I think that what conditioned me personally were the studies preceding the introduction on the market of Alvimopan, a medication used to accelerate the postoperative return of bowel function. In some of those data, the difference in hospital discharge times between study groups amounted to less than 24 h, which I thought was not clinically significant. This made me skeptical of enhanced recovery studies in general, which I realize today was narrow-minded on my part. However, in this article, these new principles were being adopted by surgeons who typically performed complex open operations rather than minimally invasive surgery. Based on their area of expertise and practices, I would not imagine they were inclined to adopt any particular perioperative measures only to accelerate postoperative recovery. And still, we could see the difference in favor of "fast track."

MD

I believe this study marked one of the earlier investigations into ERAS (Enhanced Recovery After Surgery) protocols, paving the way for numerous larger-scale studies that have since propelled these protocols into the mainstream. I think as surgeons, we naturally harbor concerns for our patients and tend to adhere closely to our own established practices. However, as we contemplate same-day colectomy, a similar conversation analogous to the one surrounding ERAS during its infancy emerges. Recent data suggests the safety and potential benefits of same-day colectomy for patients. Yet, despite supporting evidence, I remain cautious about immediate adoption. Patient selection is certainly key. Perhaps this hesitation mirrors your own experience when initially integrating ERAS protocols. It will be interesting to see how the data unfolds for same-day colectomy and what standard practices will be 20 years from now.

AM

This was among the earliest papers looking at concepts of fast-track recovery. Mayo Clinic has also published a series of papers during this era on fast track and subsequently enhanced recovery. I think our institution in general was an early adopter of these concepts, well before it became standard of care in colorectal surgery.

An important element not often highlighted is the need for widespread implementation and compliance. The care within needs to be standardized and the concepts described by Kehlet and others have been used to implement such pathways in all patients and treat all of them the same. This has been how I have tried to practice and implement ERAS in my practice, and I think it has served the patients well.

DC

I found it interesting that this was one of the early articles published in 2001 in the British Journal of Surgery, but in 1997, in the

British Journal of Anesthesia, Kehlet published some of the earliest data of what later became known as ERAS [1].

I think that ERAS not only decreased hospital stay, but it increased patient satisfaction, decreased the cost of delivering care, and paved the way for other innovative practice changes. At the risk of sounding overly philosophical, articles like these are examples of early adopters, which are the giants on whose shoulders we are sitting on. We would never be talking about same-day surgery discharges for right colectomies or ileostomy reversals if individuals such as these had not done this seminal work.

MD

Now that minimally invasive surgery is becoming more common, that adds to the benefit of enhanced recovery protocols. I think that changes it a little bit, because in this study, I think these are all open operations, right? A lot of colorectal surgery is going toward minimally invasive techniques which adds to the ability to get patients out of the hospital earlier and implement these protocols.

LS

I do not know the details of the science behind it, but I find that there is also a distinctive advantage if you implement these principles in open surgery including open complex operations. At least when I started regularly adopting ERP protocols during my career, I remember that our practices were being individually analyzed to assess the impact of ERP implementation. Among my own patients, there was a tangible advantage following protocol implementation in the laparoscopic patients, but the greatest advantage in terms of reduction of length of hospital stay occurred among open surgery patients. It was a reduction of approximately 1.7 days. And as you said Dorin, the patients were happier; they were not feeling they were being kicked out of the hospital.

AM

The next iteration of ERAS is really moving more of what we do to ambulatory surgery. There will always be an element of our practice that needs hospitals. But these concepts of hospital at home and moving less acute patients out of the inpatient setting are gaining steam.

DC

What about carbohydrate loading? Have you found it to make a difference? It is sometimes packaged with ERAS.

MD

I do not find the data in support of it particularly robust. If the evidence were compelling, my stance might be different. However, as it stands, I do not believe it justifies the financial and time investment required for implementation or strong advocacy, especially with data that lacks substantial strength.

AM

Agree. The data is more variable, but there is some support for it. I think barriers remain cost and patient compliance.

LS

I would be okay with it, but I have not been fanatic about it, and what I have read has not been so convincing to me. Where I used to work, we tried to implement it at some point, and there was a big barrier because it was something that was largely not covered by insurance. And so, it is like you have this initiative, but most of the patients were not willing to buy this on their own, and so it just could not work. Perhaps this has changed now.

Reference

1. Kehlet H. Multimodal approach to control postoperative pathophysiology and rehabilitation. Br J Anaesth. 1997;78(5):606–17.

Laparoscopic Lavage for Complicated Diverticulitis

32

Vennix S, Musters GD, Mulder IM, Swank HA, Consten EC, Belgers EH, van Geloven AA, Gerhards MF, Govaert MJ, van Grevenstein WM, Hoofwijk AG, Kruyt PM, Nienhuijs SW, Boermeester MA, Vermeulen J, van Dieren S, Lange JF, Bemelman WA; Ladies trial collaborators. Laparoscopic peritoneal lavage or sigmoidectomy for perforated diverticulitis with purulent peritonitis: a multicentre, parallel-group, randomised, open-label trial. Lancet. 2015;386(10000):1269–77.

Abstract

Background: Case series suggest that laparoscopic peritoneal lavage might be a promising alternative to sigmoidectomy in patients with perforated diverticulitis. We aimed to assess the superiority of laparoscopic lavage compared with sigmoidectomy in patients with purulent perforated diverticulitis, with respect to overall long-term morbidity and mortality.

Methods: We did a multicenter, parallel-group, randomized, open-label trial in 34 teaching hospitals and eight academic hospitals in Belgium, Italy, and the Netherlands (the Ladies trial). The Ladies trial is split into two groups: the LOLA group comparing laparoscopic lavage with sigmoidectomy and the DIVA group comparing Hartmann's procedure with sigmoidectomy plus primary anastomosis. The DIVA section of this trial is still underway, but here we report the results of the LOLA section. Patients with puru-

© The Author(s), under exclusive license to Springer Nature Switzerland AG 2025

D. Colibaseanu et al., *Essential Articles in Colorectal Surgery*, https://doi.org/10.1007/978-3-031-77745-5_32

lent perforated diverticulitis were enrolled for LOLA, excluding patients with fecal peritonitis, aged older than 85 years, with high-dose steroid use (≥20 mg daily), and hemodynamic instability. Patients were randomly assigned (2:1:1; stratified by age [<60 years vs. ≥60 years]) using secure online computer randomization to laparoscopic lavage, Hartmann's procedure, or primary anastomosis in a parallel design after diagnostic laparoscopy. Patients were analyzed according to a modified intention-to-treat principle and were followed up after the index operation at least once in the outpatient setting and after sigmoidoscopy and stoma reversal, according to local protocols. The primary endpoint was a composite endpoint of major morbidity and mortality within 12 months. This trial is registered with ClinicalTrials.gov, number NCT01317485.

Findings: Between July 1, 2010, and Feb 22, 2013, 90 patients were randomly assigned in the LOLA section of the Ladies trial when the study was terminated by the data and safety monitoring board because of an increased event rate in the lavage group. Two patients were excluded for protocol violations. The primary endpoint occurred in 30 (67%) of 45 patients in the lavage group and 25 (60%) of 42 patients in the sigmoidectomy group (odds ratio 1.28, 95% CI 0.54–3.03, $p = 0.58$). By 12 months, four patients had died after lavage and six patients had died after sigmoidectomy ($p = 0.43$).

Interpretation: Laparoscopic lavage is not superior to sigmoidectomy for the treatment of purulent perforated diverticulitis.

LS

When laparoscopic lavage was proposed, it was advocated as the new and improved minimally invasive treatment for sigmoid diverticulitis complicated by purulent peritonitis. Several retrospective studies indicated excellent results, emphasizing the avoidance of both sigmoid resection and stoma creation. A systematic review published in 2010 including 231 patients from 11 studies and two case reports indicated a success rate in controlling abdominal and systemic sepsis of almost 96% [1]. This degree of enthusiasm was certainly tamed in subsequent years by the results of studies having a more rigorous design. Throughout this time, I remained hesitant to adopt this approach because often times patients with purulent peritonitis in my workplace had severe associated comorbidities and I felt they would not have the reserve to tolerate treatment failures and recurrent or persistent abdominal sepsis following initial laparoscopic lavage. A recent study combining the data from the LOLA and the SCANDIV [2] trials identified smoking and corticosteroid use as independent factors associated with failure of laparoscopic lavage, defined as morbidity requiring general anesthesia (Clavien-Dindo IIIb or higher) within 90 days [3]. Other studies have identified other independent factors associated with laparo-scopic lavage failure including ASA grade over 3, immunosup-pression, increased BMI, and higher Mannheim Peritonitis Index score. The subpopulation at risk of failure is exactly the subpopu-lation that I feel could poorly tolerate failure. Recognizing that laparoscopic lavage can benefit some patients, should such high-risk subpopulation be selected away from it? This was even more the case after I read the results of this prospective randomized trial. I actually saw Dr. Bemelman presenting the trial results at a conference before I read the article so that I already knew some of the substantive content. The Data Monitoring and Safety Board had interrupted the trial given an alarmingly high rate of reoperations in the lavage group. This trial was supposed to test laparoscopic lavage as the future treatment options of choice in this patient population. To be honest, other trials have been con-ducted, and the results have been mixed. The investigators of the DILALA trial remain proponents of laparoscopic lavage based on their own randomized trial results [4]. In the early days of laparoscopic lavage, I was confused on the ideal approach to the perforation area. Should we dissect the perforated sigmoid colon and attempt laparoscopic closure? Could this aggravate the sep-sis? Were some of the early successes reported in the literature actual cases of Hinchey 2 treated with laparoscopic lavage in the absence of available interventional radiology service to perform percutaneous abscess drainage? In all the prospective random-ized trials, the selection of Hinchey III patients was accurately monitored, and no attempts were made to dissect around the area of perforation. Laparoscopic rinsing of the entire abdominal cavity with saline solution was associated with the placement of one or two drains around the perforation area. This has at least clarified and simplified any doubts on surgical technique. The ultimate results of the LOLA trial and even more the 3-year results indicated that laparoscopic lavage could have a role. My personal hesitation to embrace laparoscopic lavage revolves around patient selection and the discomfort of waiting for a severe complication to occur in the first days postoperatively when in comparison I feel I would not be so anxious after a resection. A total of 45% of patients in the LOLA trial eventually required surgery, but only some of this proportion was due to recurrent episodes of diverticulitis which we could perhaps view as another episode of diverticulitis which could occur in patients who have not had surgery yet.

References

1. Toorenvliet BR, Swank H, Schoones JW, Hamming JF, Bemelman WA. Laparoscopic peritoneal lavage for perforated colonic diverticulitis: a systematic review. Colorectal Dis. 2010;12(9):862–7.
2. Schultz JK, Yaqub S, Wallon C, Blecic L, Forsmo HM, Folkesson J, Buchwald P, Körner H, Dahl FA, Øresland T; SCANDIV Study Group. Laparoscopic Lavage vs Primary Resection for Acute Perforated Diverticulitis: the SCANDIV Randomized Clinical Trial. JAMA. 2015;314(13):1364–75.
3. Azhar N, Lambrichts D, Lange J, Yaqub S, Øresland T, Schultz J, Bemelman W, Buchwald P. Laparoscopic lavage for Hinchey III perforated diverticulitis: factors for treatment failure in two randomized clinical trials. Br J Surg. 2023;110(7):846–51.
4. Kohl A, Rosenberg J, Bock D, Bisgaard T, Skullman S, Thornell A, Gehrman J, Angenete E, Haglind E. Two-year results of the randomized clinical trial DILALA comparing laparoscopic lavage with resection as treatment for perforated diverticulitis. Br J Surg. 2018;105(9):1128–34.

Discussion

DC

At the time this study on laparoscopic lavage came out, I was toward the end of my training, and I did use this a couple times, but I had to go back and perform a Hartmann's in both cases. And so, I decided to then wait longer and see what the data coalesces to, and once it did, it became clear to me that this was probably not a great way to go.

MD

Yes, this technique gained popularity during my residency when I was a PGY-2/3. We had a young attending who was really enthusiastic about it, who attempted this approach on a few occasions, but it often did not yield favorable results, often requiring take-back to the operating room.

I think the challenge lies in accurately distinguishing between purulent and feculent peritonitis solely based on a CT scan. Oftentimes, when encountering an abscess in the operating room, extensive manipulation is required to access and drain the area of sepsis. While the technique has proven effective for some patients, particularly in avoiding stomas or further surgery altogether, there remains the concern for significant immediate postoperative morbidity and criteria for patient selection.

Although patients in the laparoscopic lavage group did require more acute preoperative intervention, 52% were successfully treated with this technique. So, while laparoscopic lavage does work in some scenarios, it is challenging to predict which patients will benefit. I share your perspective that it is not something I currently offer in my practice.

For those who do offer laparoscopic lavage, transparency with patients is essential. Patients must be informed of the elevated risk of reoperation and persistent intra-abdominal sepsis and the need for vigilant monitoring to ensure timely intervention if complications arise.

LS

I agree. I think it works for some patients. What I find difficult to conceive is how you practice surgery when you have a high percentage of patients who will get sick and could get sick at night or during a weekend when you are not immediately there. I have never done it. I went through the phase of excitement when reading papers preceding the LOLA trial, and there was a large number of retrospective studies which indicated that lavage was better than what we were doing that far, either Hartmann or resection with anastomosis and diversion. This paper was important to me because it was very well designed and corroborated our doubts about it. I admired the science behind it and the rigor in conducting the trial and the fact that it had to be interrupted, because of safety concerns in the lavage arm, but in follow-up, the two study groups ended up being more comparable. When the longer-term studies are assessed, there are groups which are more enthusiastic about it than perhaps the LOLA investigators. So, there are some differences, but to me, the science convinced me that it can work, but it also gives me an idea of what happens when lavage does not work, which is what gives me pause in adopting this technique.

MD

The SCANDIV trial, which followed, also yielded similar results with higher rates of deep surgical site infection and unplanned reoperation in the laparoscopic lavage group. With two randomized controlled studies showing similar short-term complications with laparoscopic lavage, in my opinion, this is not a procedure that should be routinely offered.

DC

I guess washouts are a great thing to do on a Friday, and then, you leave and let your partners sort it out.

LS

Maybe in some practices lavage can work better or maybe I was never close to somebody who taught me that in practice. Until I find that person or until one of my partners comes to me and says, "I went and learned this, we can do it in that way now," I think it will be hard to implement it.

Laparoscopic vs. Open Sigmoidectomy for Diverticulitis

33

Klarenbeek BR, Veenhof AA, Bergamaschi R, van der Peet DL, van den Broek WT, de Lange ES, Bemelman WA, Heres P, Lacy AM, Engel AF, Cuesta MA. Laparoscopic sigmoid resection for diverticulitis decreases major morbidity rates: a randomized control trial: short-term results of the Sigma Trial. Ann Surg. 2009;249(1):39–44.

Abstract

Background: No randomized controlled trial has compared laparoscopic sigmoid resection (LSR) to open sigmoid resection (OSR) for symptomatic diverticulitis of the sigmoid colon. This study tested the hypothesis that LSR is associated with decreased postoperative complication rates as compared with OSR.

Methods: This was a prospective, multicenter, double-blind, parallel-arm, randomized controlled trial. Eligible patients were randomized to either LSR or OSR. Endpoints included postoperative mortality, and complications were classified as major and minor. The generator of the allocation sequence was separated from the executor. Blinding was ensured using an opaque wound dressing to cover the abdomen. Symptomatic diverticulitis of the sigmoid colon was defined as recurrent disease Hinchey I, IIa, IIb, symptomatic stricture, or severe rectal bleeding. The decision to discharge patients was made by independent physicians blind to the allocation sequence. Data were analyzed according to the intention-to-treat principle.

Results: From 2002 to 2006, 104 patients were randomized in five centers. All patients underwent the allocated intervention. Fifty-two LSR patients were comparable to 52 OSR patients for gender, age, BMI, ASA grade, comorbid conditions, previous abdominal surgery, and indication for surgery. LSR took longer ($P = 0.0001$) but caused less blood loss ($P = 0.033$). Conversion rate was 19.2%. Mortality rate was 1%. There were significantly more major complications in OSR patients (9.6% vs. 25.0%; $P = 0.038$). Minor complication rates were similar (LSR 36.5% vs. OSR 38.5%; $P = 0.839$). LSR patients had less pain (Visual Analog Scale 1.6; $P = 0.0003$), systemic analgesia requirement ($P = 0.029$), and returned home earlier ($P = 0.046$). The short form-36 questionnaire showed significantly better quality of life for LSR.

Conclusions: LSR was associated with a 15.4% reduction in major complication rates, less pain, improved quality of life, and shorter hospitalization at the cost of a longer operating time.

LS

This landmark trial demonstrated improved outcome after laparoscopic vs. open surgery and contributed at the time of its publication to corroborate the preferential use of the laparoscopic approach for sigmoid diverticular disease. Perhaps, the most impressive aspect of this trial was that the investigators applied the principles of double-blind design as strictly as one could imagine for a surgical study. Both patients and treating caregivers were blinded to the allocated treatment by placing a large dressing on top of the abdomen (its photograph is included in the original publication) so that the patient could not see any incisions which could suggest either a laparoscopic or an open operation. Patients were ultimately asked to guess the surgical approach used on themselves as part of the study, and 58% of patients undergoing open surgery correctly guessed vs. 32% after laparoscopic surgery, which however was not statistically significant. On the other hand, this trial identified a statistically significant difference in morbidity favoring the laparoscopic approach, a difference which could not be confirmed by two subsequent randomized trials [1, 2].

More importantly, there was also a significant decrease in the length of hospital stay associated with the laparoscopic group, which was subsequently confirmed by another trial [1] applying the same principles of blinded treatment allocation. The reduction in length of hospital stay aligned with the randomized data which were being published during the same period on laparoscopic vs. open colectomy for cancer, which further cemented minimally invasive surgery as the preferential approach in the elective treatment of sigmoid diverticulitis. In this time and age, the debate has perhaps shifted on whether robotic surgery is preferable to laparoscopic surgery which might render this trial at least in the future obsolete. In a systematic review and meta-analysis on 15 articles including over 3711 robotic procedures, robotic surgery was associated with reduced conversion rates compared with laparoscopic surgery, while postoperative morbidity was similar [3]. While the use of robotic surgery is increasing in the United States, in other countries, laparoscopic surgery remains highly prevalent. For example, in a recent multicenter French national cohort study on sigmoid diverticulitis treated surgically, 88% of the procedures were performed laparoscopically [4]. A randomized trial comparing laparoscopic and robotic sigmoidectomy as elective treatment for sigmoid diverticulitis would seem the logical sequela of the Sigma trial from a strictly scientific perspective but remains unlikely to be designed and implemented. It is more probable that surgeon preferences and market forces within different healthcare systems will play a greater role in determining the prevalent minimally invasive approach in various parts of the world.

References

1. Gervaz P, Inan I, Perneger T, Schiffer E, Morel P. A prospective, randomized, single-blind comparison of laparoscopic versus open sigmoid colectomy for diverticulitis. Ann Surg. 2010;252(1):3–8.
2. Raue W, Paolucci V, Asperger W, Albrecht R, Büchler MW, Schwenk W; LAPDIV-CAMIC Trial Group. Laparoscopic sigmoid resection for diverticular disease has no advantages

over open approach: midterm results of a randomized controlled trial. Langenbecks Arch Surg. 2011;396(7):973–80.

3. Sabbagh C, Beyer-Berjot L, Ouaissi M, Zerbib P, Bridoux V, Manceau G, Karoui M, Panis Y, Buscail E, Venara A, Khaoudy I, Gaillard M, Ortega-Deballon P, Viennet M, Thobie A, Menahem B, Eveno C, Bonnel C, Mabrut JY, Badic B, Godet C, Eid Y, Duchalais E, Lakkis Z, Cotte E, Laforest A, Defourneaux V, Maggiori L, Rebibo L, Christou N, Talal A, Mege D, Bonnamy C, Germain A, Mauvais F, Tresallet C, Ahmed O, Regimbeau JM, Roudie J, Laurent A, Trilling B, Bertrand M, Massalou D, Romain B, Tranchart H, Giger U, Dejardin O, Pellegrin A, Alves A; French Surgical Association. Risk factors for severe morbidity and definitive stoma after elective surgery for sigmoid diverticulitis: a multicenter national cohort study. Tech Coloproctol. 2024;28(1):34.

4. Larkins K, Mohan H, Apte SS, Chen V, Rajkomar A, Larach JT, Smart P, Heriot A, Warrier S. A systematic review and meta-analysis of robotic resections for diverticular disease. Colorectal Dis. 2022;24(10):1105–16. https://doi.org/10.1111/codi.16227. Epub 2022 Aug 9.

Discussion

DC

This study was done over 15 years ago, and it had a lot of value at the time. It compared open and laparoscopic surgery in colorectal benign disease focusing on mortality, morbidity, and quality of life. By this time, we already had some data that laparoscopic surgery was likely beneficial, but no prospective, randomized, double-blind trial had been done yet. Not unsurprisingly, they excluded previous low laparotomies and acute diverticulitis. Their final outcomes published in 2010 found benefits favoring the laparoscopic approach (15.4% morbidity reduction), but in the long term, there were no differences. Even the SF-36 questionnaire showed similar long-term (after 6 months) quality of life, though the short term favored the laparoscopic approach.

MD

Yes, I think part of that, too, is that I think a lot of general surgeons do more diverticular disease, and they may do cancer surgery and they may not be as inclined to approach these cases laparoscopically. A lot of diverticular disease cases which I guess this study mentions are elective, but in the urgent setting, surgery is generally done more open than in a minimally invasive fashion. At the time of this trial, the inclusion criteria were also different from the diverticulitis presentations we really operate on now. For example, the authors included patients who were under the age of 50 with one diverticulitis episode. And now we have moved away from the idea that diverticulitis is a progressive disease and just being under 50 years old and having one uncomplicated disease episode is no longer really a strong indication for surgery. And then they included patients that were older than, 50 with just with two uncomplicated disease episodes, and again, these are not exactly the criteria we use today. I think now we are really operating more on complicated diseases, for example, fistulizing disease or stricture. I find that the breakdown of patients with more complicated disease was not exactly clear in the study, but I think that the patient population we are operating on now is more complicated than the patients who were included in this study, which may contribute to the lack of minimally invasive surgery done for diverticular disease now, perhaps compared to the population that was studied here.

AM

Here is another trial that shows the benefits of minimally invasive surgery over open. What is interesting to me is that when detractors of robotics compare it to laparoscopy, they often cite that short- and long-term outcomes are no different. Yet here is a study that is promoting laparoscopy, yet the long-term outcomes are no different than open surgery. The true comparison when considering robotics should be to open surgery, not laparoscopy.

LS

As far as the penetration of laparoscopic versus robotic surgery, I think that this is also a study that does not come from the United States. I think in Europe the use of robotic surgery is still less common than in the United States. Your points are well taken with respect to the possible causes why robotic surgery or even laparoscopic surgery are not more used in the US. I think that in Europe and elsewhere in the world, the healthcare environment is very different in terms of costs, reimbursement, etc. which might be one of the factors responsible for the low prevalence of robotic surgery there and renders direct comparisons of surgical techniques more difficult.

The Advent of Ligation of the Intersphincteric Tract to Treat Anal Fistulas

34

Rojanasakul A, Pattanaarun J, Sahakitrungruang C, Tantiphlachiva K. Total anal sphincter saving technique for fistula-in-ano; the ligation of intersphincteric fistula tract. J Med Assoc Thai. 2007;90:581–6.

Abstract

Objective: To describe a new technique for fistula-in-ano surgery aimed at total sphincter preservation and evaluate the preliminary results concerning non-healing and intact anal function.

Material and Method: A prospective observational study in 18 fistula-in-ano patients treated by ligation of intersphincteric fistula tract (LIFT) technique, from January to June 2006.

Results: Fistula-in-ano in 17 patients healed primarily (94.4%). There was one non-healing case (5.6%). The mean healing time was 4 weeks. None had disturbances in clinical anal continence.

Conclusion: The early outcome of the LIFT technique is quite impressive. Results warrant a larger study with long-term evaluation. This technique has the potential to become a viable option for fistula-in-ano surgery.

© The Author(s), under exclusive license to Springer Nature Switzerland AG 2025
D. Colibaseanu et al., *Essential Articles in Colorectal Surgery*,
https://doi.org/10.1007/978-3-031-77745-5_34

LS

I did not read this article before I started using the ligation of the intersphincteric tract (LIFT) in my practice, but this is the original publication which deserves the credit. I knew of Dr. Rojanasakul through colleagues and especially through articles on LIFT published in American journals and attended his presentations on this technique. The description of the technique made logical sense, and I was encouraged by witnessed results in the hands of colleagues, which ultimately won my initial hesitation to immediately embrace the new and bold. I feel that the acceptance of LIFT as a feasible surgical approach was hampered in part by the natural resistance to change but also suffered from an additional modicum of diffidence toward what does not come from North America, Australia, or Europe. Good surgery can be practiced all over the world, and innovative ideas can surely originate outside of the Anglo-Western countries. This has been the case with LIFT. A number of reports from different institutions over the world have confirmed that LIFT is an acceptable approach to treat anal fistula. Its success rate is very variable, between 47% and 95% in one review of 26 studies [1]. Arguably, LIFT has positioned itself as the main alternative to mucosal advancement flap for higher fistulas involving a substantial portion of the sphincter muscle. Mucosal advancement flap can be technically difficult, and sometimes, recurrence can lead to worse fistula symptoms when compared with the original fistula, especially in Crohn's disease. The preference for one technique over the other also depends on individual experiences and training. A recent prospective randomized trial has indicated better results after LIFT [2], but the literature has generally not indicated a clear superiority of one technique over the other. I personally prefer LIFT to a mucosal advancement flap, and I did notice that a recurrence after LIFT is often in the form of a more superficial intersphincteric fistula, which can be successfully treated with a secondary fistulotomy [3]. This typically does not compromise continence. The original LIFT technique was described for idiopathic fistula-in-ano. However, LIFT has also been successfully used for Crohn's disease, which is an extension of its original indication, although still controversial. The Cedars Sinai group has reported a long-term healing rate of 65%. Smoking was associated with a significantly increased risk of failure, while active proctitis did not quite reach statistical significance [4].

References

1. Sirany AM, Nygaard RM, Morken JJ. The ligation of the inter-sphincteric fistula tract procedure for anal fistula: a mixed bag of results. Dis Colon Rectum. 2015;58(6):604–12.
2. Kumar P, Sarthak S, Singh PK, Mishra TS, Sasmal PK. Ligation of intersphincteric fistulous tract vs endorectal advancement flap for high-type fistula in ano: a randomized controlled trial. J Am Coll Surg. 2023;236(1):27–35.
3. Tan KK, Tan IJ, Lim FS, Koh DC, Tsang CB. The anatomy of failures following the ligation of intersphincteric tract technique for anal fistula: a review of 93 patients over 4 years. Dis Colon Rectum. 2011;54(11):1368–72.
4. Wood T, Truong A, Mujukian A, Zaghiyan K, Fleshner P. Increasing experience with the LIFT procedure in Crohn's disease patients with complex anal fistula. Tech Coloproctol. 2022;26(3):205–12.

Discussion

MD

I feel LIFT is a great technique which allowed us to offer patients an additional surgical alternative to mucosal advancement flap. It is especially helpful in situations where a flap has failed. In my practice, I actually prefer a LIFT over a flap if possible.

LS

I also prefer a LIFT in general.

MD

Maybe it's just my technique with the flap, but I have better success with the LIFT. As reported in the literature, in my experience with LIFT, if a fistula recurs, I have often been able to perform a subsequent intersphincteric fistulotomy to address the recurrence. Unlike with a mucosal advancement flap, the fistula track can be much smaller after LIFT failure.

I think by the time I finished my training, it was widely accepted that LIFT was an acceptable alternative, either flap or LIFT. But you guys may have more experience with the initial acceptance of LIFT when this paper was written.

LS

I feel it was viewed as an oddity because it was coming from outside of the Western world, and it took longer time to become accepted. But now it is highly regarded as an accepted standard of care. The Cedar Sinai group has published results of LIFT done in patients with Crohn's disease as well.

I've also used LIFT for some patients with Crohn's who have single transphincteric fistulas. I use the criteria similarly to hemorrhoidectomy or surgery for anal fissure in this patient population. If there is no active disease in the rectum, I do mention risks of healing which could derive from Crohn's disease, but I do feel that it is an option that can be offered. Of course, in looking at all comers with Crohn's disease, it is more likely to have synchronous rectal inflammation and/or complex perianal disease, with multiple branching fistulas etc. which would be contraindications to LIFT.

Michelle, I echo your words to the letter. I also feel that it's more difficult for me to do a flap and manage a possible failure. I have been referred to patients who I did LIFT after a flap had already failed elsewhere. In those cases, I felt a different operation with a dissection conducted through different planes was going to be easier and more successful, so I became more comfortable with this technique. I also didn't know about this original article. I think it is the article that we need to quote to give credit to those who were the first to conceive and present this technique. I came to know about the group that published this indirectly because where I used to work (Cleveland Clinic, OH) one of the coauthors of the original paper was at some point an international fellow in colorectal surgery, and so that's how I came to know the group. Honestly, I don't think that I can reproduce the results of that group. A LIFT can fail, and the fistula can recur, but again as you pointed out, there is a subset of failures that result in an inter-sphincteric fistula, which can be comfortably treated with fisto-lotomy so that we can basically achieve secondary success.

DC

The success of the LIFT procedure varies and, from what I can tell, is a little bit less successful in the US. It seems like obesity and young age are associated with decreased success rates. Thus, I find myself doing rectal advancement flaps at least as often as LIFTs, and certainly more commonly in overweight individuals, and so I am skewed toward doing LIFT procedures in thinner individuals. What I found interesting in more recent articles, in cases where LIFT failed initially, reinterventions were remarkably successful (not necessarily another LIFT), which is encouraging. I would say I'm probably the odd man out with this because I'm more likely to do a flap than a LIFT.

LS

What are your criteria besides obesity to decide on flap versus LIFT?

DC

Though advancement flaps are associated with better outcomes in higher fistulas, I find that reaching to do a transanal advancement flap in a high fistula can be more difficult. As noted, I'm more skewed in my own preference towards transanal flaps, but I would probably do a LIFT first in an individual in whom I think I would have a hard time getting to the fistula transanally.

LS

One thing about flaps that I have not seen in LIFTs at least so far is that I feel that the failure of a flap can lead to fistula symptoms that are worse than the original symptoms. And that is something that really gave me pause in terms of favoring flaps over LIFTs, where I have seen that in case of failure, the patient goes back to the original symptoms or has a more superficial recurrent intersphincteric fistula amenable to fistulotomy, as Michelle mentioned earlier.

DC

Have you guys ever heard about the LIFT-plug technique?

LS

I heard of it but have no experience.

DC

This is in the Annals of Surgery out of China with a staggering number of patients, 235 randomized to either LIFT or LIFT with plug, 117 or so patients in each group [1]. They found that the LIFT+plug technique was more successful.

MD

It's different than a bio lift, where a piece of biologic material is inserted for either scaffolding or as a mesh in the intersphincteric space.

DC

They used porcine-derived tissue. Again, it is used in a population that is probably thinner than our Western patients, and even though their technique is published, I do not know if I would be able to replicate its results.

Reference

1. Han JG, Wang ZJ, Zheng Y, Chen CW, Wang XQ, Che XM, Song WL, Cui JJ. Ligation of intersphincteric fistula tract vs ligation of the intersphincteric fistula tract plus a bioprosthetic anal fistula plug procedure in patients with transsphincteric anal fistula: early results of a multicenter prospective randomized trial. Ann Surg. 2016;264(6):917–22.

Rectal Polyp, Risk of Malignancy, and the Limitations of Magnetic Resonance Staging

35

Penman D, Keogh A, Ahmed S, Ahmed S, Farrell C, Andrews T, Javed A, Sarkar S. Substratifying the risk of covert malignancy in significant rectal polyps: outcomes from a specialist multidisciplinary team (MDT). Colorectal Dis. 2024;26(6):1145–52.

Abstract

Aim: A treatment strategy for patients with a significant polyp or early colon cancer (SPECC) of the rectum presents a challenge due to the significant rate of covert malignancy and lack of standardized assessment. For this reason, NICE recommends multidisciplinary meetings to improve outcomes. The primary aim of this study was to report the performance of our specialist early rectal cancer (SERC) multidisciplinary team (MDT) in correctly substratifying the risk of cancer and to discuss the limitations of staging investigations in those patients with "poor outcomes."

Method: This was a retrospective review of patients referred to our SERC MDT from 2014 to 2019. Lesions were assigned by the MDT to three pre-resection categories (low, intermediate, high) according to the risk of covert malignancy. Resection method and final histology were compared to the pre-resection categories.

Results: Of 350 SPECC lesions, 174 were assessed as low-risk, 108 intermediate-risk, and 68 high-risk. The cancer incidence was 4.8%, 8.3%, and 53%, respectively (15.5% overall). Eight lesions were categorized as low-risk but following piece-

© The Author(s), under exclusive license to Springer Nature Switzerland AG 2025

D. Colibaseanu et al., *Essential Articles in Colorectal Surgery*, https://doi.org/10.1007/978-3-031-77745-5_35

meal resection were found to be malignant. Five lesions, three of which were categorized as high-risk, were ultimately benign following conventional surgery. One pT1sm1 cancer, removed by anterior resection, may have been treated by local excision.

Conclusion: A total of 83% of malignant polyps were triaged to an en bloc resection technique and surgical resection avoided for nearly all benign lesions. However, 12 patients from this cohort were deemed to have a poor outcome because of miscategorization. Further comparative research is needed to establish the optimum strategy for rectal SPECC lesion assessment.

LS

This study examined the results of a dedicated unit for the treatment of large polypoid lesions of the rectum. The primary goal was to compare the final histology of each specimen to the preresection risk of cancer determined by two experienced endoscopists who retrospectively reviewed the multidisciplinary team (MDT) documentation and subjectively applied a cancer risk category to each lesion: low risk, intermediate risk, and high risk. Cancer was present in 15.5% of the specimens, and its rate increased along with the risk category. The secondary goal of the study was the assessment of the accuracy of magnetic resonance imaging (MRI) and endorectal ultrasound (ERUS). A total of 20% of the 268 lesions which were either not visualized on MRI or reported as mucosal eventually turned out to be malignant. ERUS was technically unsuccessful in almost 15% of the cases. Among the patients having technically successful ERUS, 8.7% of the lesions assessed as benign proved to be malignant, and 70% of the lesions indicating invasion on ERUS were ultimately benign on surgical pathology. The very existence of a dedicated unit which evaluated and decided through MDT meetings on the management of these lesions is impressive. This only partially overlaps with the traditional tumor board for the discussion of rectal cancer cases. For example, the regular inclusion of endoscopists in the MDT, which would be unusual in the United States, could optimize decision-making. The acknowledgment of a uniform referral pattern to a dedicated unit might minimize those occurrences when patients are discussed only after they have already undergone endoscopic excision, and surgeons could not participate in the initial decision-making. Importantly, this study confirms that MRI of the pelvis, the fundamental imaging modality for loco-regional staging of rectal cancer, remains inaccurate in distinguishing between benign and malignant rectal lesions. This adds to the known limitations in assessing the T staging of known malignant lesions, which were excluded from this study. ERUS might contribute useful information in an individual case but remains largely unreliable especially if used in isolation. Considering the ongoing limitations of available imaging techniques, some surgeons have proposed that clinically large benign polypoid lesions should undergo initial local excision without prior imaging [1]. Local excision remains necessary in at least a proportion of cases. After that, a subset of patients can still require completion proctectomy. This is arguably more difficult and associated with worse outcomes than upfront proctectomy. A systematic review on 16 studies involving 353 patients indicated that completion proctectomy following transanal local excision resulted in incomplete mesorectal fascia in almost 25% of cases, and the abdomino-perineal resection rate was 23.2%. These data were admittedly incomplete and of low quality but indicated a tendency toward an increased risk of permanent colostomy and poor specimen quality [2]. Although more recent experiences have indicated similar outcomes when comparing completion proctectomy after local excision and primary resection [3, 4], these data underscore the importance of careful decision-making in the management of these still challenging lesions.

References

1. Lee L, Arbel L, Albert MR, Atallah SB, Hill J, Monson JRT. Radiologic evaluation of clinically benign rectal neoplasms may not be necessary before local excision. Dis Colon Rectum. 2018;61(10):1163–9.

2. Zinicola R, Nascimbeni R, Cirocchi R, Gagliardi G, Cracco N, Giuffrida M, Pedrazzi G, Binda GA. The impact of transanal local excision of early rectal cancer on completion rectal resection without neoadjuvant chemoradiotherapy: a systematic review. Tech Coloproctol. 2021;25(9):997–1010.
3. Levic Souzani K, Bulut O, Kuhlmann TP, Gögenur I, Bisgaard T. Completion total mesorectal excision following transanal endoscopic microsurgery does not compromise outcomes in patients with rectal cancer. Surg Endosc. 2022;36(2):1181–90.
4. Burghgraef TA, Rutgers ML, Leijtens JWA, Tuyman JB, Consten ECJ, Hompes R. Completion total mesorectal excision: a case-matched comparison with primary resection. Ann Surg Open. 2023;4(3):e327.

Discussion

DC

I did not understand it very well, to be honest. I read both the paper and the comments. But what I can tell is that ideally we would have a dedicated team that would evaluate these polyps with both EUS and MRI, a team with sufficient experience, but we just do not have that. EUS is rarely used nowadays, at least for us, and we depend so much on the MRI. This is still an area with significant uncharted territory.

LS

The reason for selecting this study was that it is a contemporary series which includes ample use of MR for staging but still demonstrates limitations in establishing an accurate preoperative diagnosis with a persistent and relatively high rate of inaccurate diagnosis. And to reconnect to some of the discussions that we had in the past with respect to local excision of rectal cancer, we are still faced with a situation where, despite MR being the preferred and fundamental test for loco-regional staging, this is yet frequently inaccurate to reassure about the absence of malignancy or vice versa in many cases, and the lesion can be read as a cancer, sometimes even a locally advanced cancer, when it is in fact a large adenoma which has happened to me a few times. Without a biopsy-proven cancer, I feel a proctectomy is not warranted, and I perform a local excision which often reveals that the lesion is benign. There is one reference related to this from Advent Health Orlando where the authors did not use MR frequently, unlike in the article we are discussing, and they basically questioned the use of any staging studies for large, clinically benign rectal lesions. They felt that in most cases, it is necessary to just locally excise the lesion, establish the diagnosis on the specimen pathology, and take it from there. At the same time, I feel that if you do this systematically, you can find yourself in certain situations where you could have done a definitive procedure for cancer, which is done with wider margins, and you could predispose yourself to a potentially much more difficult completion proctectomy, depending also on the location of the mass. If it is a posterior mass completely covered by mesorectum, the rectal dissection might not be altered, but in case of a lesion located for example distally with minimal mesorectal coverage, the dissection planes can become distorted because of the previous local excision, and even an intraoperative perforation could occur through the local excision defect or suture line. A completion proctectomy following local excision is at times inevitable but should be avoided if possible in favor of definitive local excision or initial and definitive proctectomy.

DC

I found it worrisome that in patients who did have a local excision and had cancer, a significant proportion, almost one to fourth, of them had to have an abdomino-perineal resection.

LS

Another reason why I liked this article is that it comes from a dedicated unit that assessed these lesions through multidisciplinary team meetings, which included the participation of endoscopists, and this is the kind of expertise which remains absent from the average American tumor board. Advanced endoscopists are adept at assessing complex polyps and their cancer risk through the application of accepted measurement scales such as the Paris classification and Kudo pit pattern. Their input beyond the reading of a written endoscopy report can complement other imaging modalities and optimize decision-making. Individual cases can also benefit from endorectal ultrasound, and ultimately, the work of this unit suggests that they work well together, and they could minimize the number of anterior resections for patients who had a benign lesion. All of this could ultimately offset the limitations of MR as an individual imaging study.

MD

I have had the same experience with endorectal ultrasound and, I think as in this study, MRI, because the MRI is so poor in determining T1 vs. T2 staging and certainly in assessing mucosal lesions. In this study, if the MR was showing a bulky tumor, obviously they were not going to be proceeding with an endoscopic reception. But I have not found that endorectal ultrasound has been particularly helpful in that it generally will overcall lesions. I have had many large polyps which were read as T2, even T3 cancers, but ultimately did not have a pathologic diagnosis of cancer like you were saying, Luca. So, I think that until we get better imaging to help us assess those smaller mucosal lesions, T1 and T2 transanal excision of these lesions is required to establish a diagnosis before determining definitive treatment.

LS

In practice, which is an aspect that perhaps was not the specific focus of this particular article, when I see a reading of T3 on MR or there are some synchronous lymph nodes which could be malignant, raising the possibility of chemotherapy and/or radiotherapy, I have also repeated endoscopy with biopsies rather than immediately venturing into local excision, especially when I feel that endoscopically it looks like a cancer. I prefer to go through this extra step understanding that biopsies could be still benign thus requiring a subsequent local excision, but sometimes I have been successful in obtaining an invasive cancer diagnosis. In that case and despite the ongoing MR limitations which you were alluding to, I find that the discussion of a biopsy-proven malignancy and the decision on its most appropriate management plan become a little clearer.

Management of Positive Air Leak Test After Left-Sided Colorectal Anastomosis

36

Ricciardi R, Roberts PL, Marcello PW, Hall JF, Read TE, Schoetz DJ. Anastomotic leak testing after colorectal resection: what are the data? Arch Surg. 2009;144(5):407–11; discussion 411–2.

Abstract

Objective: To determine the value of anastomotic leak testing of left-sided colorectal anastomoses.

Design: Cohort analysis.

Setting: Subspecialty practice at a tertiary care facility.

Patients: Consecutive subjects were selected from a prospective colorectal database of 2627 patients treated between January 1, 2001, and December 31, 2007.

Intervention: Creation of left-sided colorectal anastomoses and air leak testing per surgeon preference.

Main Outcome Measures: Anastomosis type, method (handsewn vs. stapled), performance of air leak testing, repair method of anastomoses after air leak tests yielding positive results, and development of postoperative clinical leak.

Results: A total of 998 left-sided colorectal anastomoses were performed without proximal diversion; 90.1% were stapled and 9.9% were handsewn. Intraoperative air leaks were noted in 65 of 825 tested anastomoses (7.9%), that is, 7.8% of stapled anastomoses and 9.5% of handsewn anastomoses. A clinical leak developed

© The Author(s), under exclusive license to Springer Nature Switzerland AG 2025

D. Colibaseanu et al., *Essential Articles in Colorectal Surgery*, https://doi.org/10.1007/978-3-031-77745-5_36

in 48 patients (4.8%). Clinical leaks were noted in 7.7% of anastomoses with positive air leak test results compared with 3.8% of anastomoses with negative air leak test results and 8.1% of all untested anastomoses ($P < 0.03$). If air leak testing yielded positive results, suture repair alone was associated with the highest rate of postoperative clinical leak compared with diversion or reanastomosis, 12.2% vs. 0% vs. 0%, respectively ($P = 0.19$).

Conclusions: Our data indicate a high rate of air leaks at air leak testing of left-sided colorectal anastomoses. In addition, the high rate of clinical leaks in untested anastomoses leads us to recommend air leak testing of all left-sided anastomoses, whether stapled or handsewn.

LS

This paper describes an unpleasant yet ultimately inevitable situation for any practicing colorectal surgery, a positive anastomotic air leak test following colorectal or ileorectal anastomosis. The authors analyzed almost 1000 ($n = 998$) of such anastomoses, over 80% of which underwent intraoperative air leak tests upon completion. These consisted of air instillation through either a proctoscope or flexible endoscope with the anastomosis under irrigation and the intestine occluded proximal to the anastomosis. None of the patients included in this study had a diverting stoma creation planned preoperatively. The rates of clinical anastomotic leak were 3.8% following a negative air leak test, 7.7% after a positive air leak test, and 8.1% when the air leak test was not performed, which was statistically significant ($p < 0.03$). When an air leak test was positive, primary suture repair alone was associated with a 12.2% (5/41) clinical anastomotic leak rate compared with no clinical anastomotic leaks after either takedown and reconstruction of the anastomosis (0/14) or stoma diversion (0/10, $p = 0.19$ in the abstract and $p = 0.41$ in the text).

It is remarkable that air leak testing is not universally performed [1, 2]. Air leak testing allows the identification of mechanical errors in the creation of the anastomosis, which if undetected are highly likely to lead to postoperative clinical anastomotic leak. Such mechanical errors can prompt reconstruction of the anastomosis when possible or the creation of a diverting stoma, both of which can significantly benefit patients. I also feel that failure to perform an air leak test may also become risky from a liability perspective, at least in the United States. There is a variety of techniques using a variable amount of air to perform air leak tests, ranging from rigid or flexible endoscopy to insufflation through a rectal catheter or through a syringe. This makes their comparison difficult. We typically perform an air leak test using a flexible sigmoidoscope to insufflate CO_2, while the pelvis is filled with saline solution or water and the bowel proximal to the anastomosis is being clamped. A flexible sigmoidoscope allows additional examination of the anastomosis for bleeding. It is possible to remove clots sitting on the anastomosis to assess whether an underlying bleeder is only temporarily covered and apply endoscopic clips as needed. Removal of a clot or residual stools can also uncover an air leak. We admittedly do not measure the CO_2 pressure elicited on the anastomosis during air leak testing and recognize that any anastomosis has an associated bursting pressure. This issue could make theoretical sense but has not been a clinical problem in our practice. Perhaps, we have not recognized it. I cannot remember a case where I felt that the very performance of the air leak test actually damaged the freshly created anastomosis. We are aware that a negative air leak test does not prevent a clinical anastomotic leak, as the present study also indicates. There was no specific information on the integrity of the anastomotic doughnuts, which is an integral part of the left-sided anastomotic testing. There are clinical situations which are germane to the theme of this article, although not strictly pertaining to its data. For example, if the positive air leak can not be technically corrected either from the abdomen and/or from the anus, for example, in a very low colorectal anastomosis in an obese male associated with an already plannned diverting ileostomy, my practice has been to place a pelvic drain to be removed before patient discharge from the hospital. Admittedly, there are no strong data to support this approach.

One aspect of this paper that I find remarkable is that it has changed my practice based on data that is not statistically significant. There are other papers assessing air leak testing and its benefits in reducing clinical anastomotic leak rates [3], but this remains the most convincing evidence on what to do if an air leak does occur. After reading this paper, I have stopped repairing the defect and repeating the air leak test until negative. I am aware the p value associated with the clinical anastomotic leak rate comparison after suture alone vs. redo anastomosis vs. diversion was not statistically significant, which means that the difference in the respective clinical leak rates could be just the result of chance. However, the numbers were small thus predisposing to type II errors, and the lack of any cases of clinical anastomotic leak was so telling that in case of a positive air leak test, I either redo the anastomosis or add a stoma diversion or both.

References

1. Song SH, Park JS, Choi GS, et al. Efficacy of air leak test in detection of anastomotic leaks after rectal excision: a retrospective case-controlled study. Ann Surg Treat Res. 2023;104(4):214–21.
2. Wu Z, van de Haar RC, Sparreboom CL, et al. Is the intraoperative air leak test effective in the prevention of colorectal anastomotic leakage? A systematic review and meta-analysis. Int J Colorectal Dis. 2016;31(8):1409–17.
3. Allaix ME, Lena A, Degiuli M, et al. Intraoperative air leak test reduces the rate of postoperative anastomotic leak: analysis of 777 laparoscopic left-sided colon resections. Surg Endosc. 2019;33(5):1592–9.

Discussion

DC

This is a Lahey Clinic study, and I found it remarkable that they were able to carry out a study with so many patients.

MD

I think there are almost 900 patients.

DC

They were able to include patients that had only attending surgeons that carried out the procedure which in my training and then subsequent practice I do not think I am able to ever do. This study supports the view that I have—that defunctionalizing an anastomosis that you have concerns with helps you deal with future complications of that anastomosis if they do occur. I think that even though the absolute percentage of leaks is small, anastomoses not tested had double the number of leaks; thus, I would always perform a leak test in a left-sided anastomosis.

MD

What do you guys do? I think for me it depends on where the anastomosis is. If it is at the sigmoid or the rectosigmoid junction, I can take it down and redo it and I am happy with it; then, I do not divert those patients. But certainly, if it needs to just be repaired, I will always divert them. And then there are some which are very low, you do not see exactly where the leak is coming from and maybe you cannot repair it, and you just divert. I have definitely been in those situations as well, but I think it depends on where the anastomosis is and the feasibility of taking it down and whether or not you would be able to take it down and create a new tension-free anastomosis, which I think really depends on the height of where it is. I think this paper was good in that it looked at a large number of patients, although it was variable with regard to where the anastomosis was, but I think it speaks to the fact that just repairing the anastomosis generally does not lead to favorable outcomes with regard to leak after that.

AM

There is more recent data than this paper which we are discussing also focusing on what to do in the setting of a positive air leak test. Similarly, the authors advocated taking the anastomosis down and redoing it, as opposed to suture repair. Admittedly, I would say that I more commonly suture repair and then divert proximally. But the decision to divert again is based on the height of the anastomosis. If the air leak is from something like a sigmoid anastomosis, then I probably would just repair or redo and repeat the leak test and, if negative, not divert them. But if it is far lower and the air leak test is positive, then again, depending on the height of the anastomosis, it may not be possible to redo it, and then, I would do a transanal repair of the defect and then divert upstream. But those are probably patients who are going to be diverted anyway, whether or not they had that positive air leak test.

LS

I find this paper very impactful on two levels. One is the value of air leak testing, which, honestly, we take for granted in the United States. And I am happy that it is so, but it has not been done all over the world, and there was a statistically significant difference between people who did have a positive test, did have a negative test, or had no test at all. The latter were associated with the worse outcome. So that is the first part, and that is what I would say the vast majority of surgeons do in the United States. The other thing that influenced me is odd because in looking at the data it was very convincing to me that I should not do an anastomotic repair of the leaking point alone, and I should either reconstruct the anastomosis or divert. And in some cases, admittedly, when it is a very low anastomosis. It might be impossible to do a repair either from below or from above. And so, in that case, I will certainly divert. Most of the time, as you pointed out, I would expect these are cases where I would divert anyway. I find it interesting that in reading the paper, it was very convincing, but suturing alone was not statistically associated with an increased rate of symptomatic leak. The absolute numbers without a significant p value were good enough for me.

DC

Have you guys ever had a situation where you would have liked to divert the anastomosis, but the patient has such a thick abdominal wall that it is very challenging to actually bring a loop ileostomy through it?

MD

I have not run into that yet, but I am sure it will happen at some point.

LS

If it is an elective case, you can see how obese the patient is in the clinic and generally develop a specific plan on where to do a stoma diversion. I think there have been cases where I felt I had to divert in urgent settings in a patient with a BMI in the 50s. In those cases, my preference is to use the right upper quadrant of the abdomen, which generally is associated with a thinner abdominal wall thickness, and then bring up the proximal transverse colon through it without trying to loop it and just create a colostomy opening from the side of the bowel and suture it flush with the skin. If possible I would prefer a matured colostomy, but given the circumstances, this has helped me. I feel in those circumstances the mesentery can be foreshortened, and passing the ileum through the thick abdominal wall can be challenging.

DC

That is a good trick. I think I am going to use it next time.

Zielinski MD, Eiken PW, Heller SF, et al. Prospective, observational validation of a multivariate small-bowel obstruction model to predict the need for operative intervention. J Am Coll Surg. 2011;212(6):1068–76.

Abstract

Background: We published previously a model predictive of the need for exploration in small-bowel obstruction. We aimed to validate and refine the model, hypothesizing that the model would be predictive, would prevent delayed management of strangulation, and would be successfully improved.

   Study Design: Data from 100 consecutive patients with small-bowel obstruction and concurrent CT were collected prospectively. New features evaluated included obstipation and the absence of colonic gas on CT.

   Results: Overall mortality was 8%. Twenty-nine patients had all 4 clinical features, 22 of whom required operative exploration (concordance index 0.75), confirming the validity of the old model. Intraperitoneal free fluid (odds ratio [OR]: 2.6, 95% CI: 1.0–6.9) and vomiting (OR: 1.5, 95% CI: 0.5–4.5) were not predictive of operative exploration; however, mesenteric edema (OR: 4.2, 95% CI: 1.1–15.8) and lack of the small-bowel feces sign were (OR: 3.5, 95% CI: 1.4–8.8). Obstipation was associated with the need for exploration (OR: 2.8, 95% CI: 1.2–6.6), but absence

© The Author(s), under exclusive license to Springer Nature Switzerland AG 2025
D. Colibaseanu et al., *Essential Articles in Colorectal Surgery*,
https://doi.org/10.1007/978-3-031-77745-5_37

of colonic gas was not. A new model was equally predictive of the need for exploration: mesenteric edema (OR: 5.6, 95% CI: 1.5–20.7), lack of the small-bowel feces sign (OR: 5.1, 95% CI: 1.9–13.6), and obstipation (OR: 3.2, 95% CI: 1.2–8.3). The concordance index for this new model was 0.77.

Conclusions: Our current prospective study validated our original model and was successfully improved. Our new model demonstrated equivalent predictive ability and was simpler to use. When all three features of the new model are present, strong consideration for early operative exploration should be entertained and may decrease the rate of missed strangulation obstructions.

LS

The management of small bowel obstruction is not a strictly colorectal surgery topic, but it is certainly a clinical presentation of numerous patients who have a history of colorectal surgery and is therefore relevant to colorectal surgeons who are called to take care of them. This is a prospective study used to validate previous retrospective work by the same group. The authors identified a model which was highly predictive of failure to respond to nonoperative management which included lack of small bowel feces sign on CT scan (presence of gas bubbles and debris within the obstructed small bowel lumen), mesenteric edema on CT scan (hazy fluid attenuation in the mesentery of the involved intestinal segment), and obstipation, defined as lack of flatus for 24 hours or longer. The CT findings included in the model imply a regular use of CT scans to evaluate patients with small bowel obstructions. This model had an accuracy of 77%. The presence of all three signs simultaneously was associated with the need for abdominal exploration in 86% of patients and a 29% rate of strangulation obstruction. In the absence of these findings, patients can be treated nonoperatively with nasogastric tube decompression and intravenous fluid rehydration. This is a very important study in that it provides a very practical set of tools to help in a clinical situation which typically requires nuanced decision-making. I have been particularly impressed over the years by the significance of the small bowel feces sign which is still considered by many surgeons as an indication of high-grade small bowel obstruction and therefore is viewed as an adverse rather than a favorable prognosticator. An adjunct to small bowel obstruction management which is not specifically addressed by this paper but was also evaluated by the same group and ultimately integrated into the model is the use of gastrografin challenge. The specific protocol varies in different institutions, but the authors recommend a mix of 100 cc of gastrografin in 50 cc of sterile water which is injected through the nasogastric tube prior to at least a 2-h period of decompression to reduce the gastrografin aspiration risk. If an abdominal X-ray taken approximately 8 h after gastrografin infusion indicates contrast in the colon or if the patient has a bowel movement/stoma function, the challenge is considered successful, thus warranting continued nonoperative management. In case of gastrografin challenge failure, operative exploration should be strongly considered as the risk of abdominal exploration during the index admission is 89% [1]. The benefits of gastrografin challenge have been confirmed in a multicenter study indicating decreased rates of abdominal exploration and decreased length of hospital stay when compared to patients who did not receive gastrografin challenge [2]. In our institution, patients with symptoms suspicious for small bowel obstruction regularly undergo CT scans of the abdomen and pelvis, and the gastrografin challenge option is also available, so I have been able to put this model into practice.

References

1. Goussous N, Eiken PW, Bannon MP, Zielinski MD. Enhancement of a small bowel obstruction model using the Gastrografin® challenge test. J Gastrointest Surg. 2013;17(1):110–6; discussion 116–7.
2. Zielinski MD, Haddad NN, Cullinane DC, et al. Multi-institutional, prospective, observational study comparing the Gastrografin challenge versus standard treatment in adhesive small bowel obstruction. J Trauma Acute Care Surg. 2017;83(1):47–54.

Discussion

DC

Martin Zielinski was my chief resident, then my attending. Great guy. It's not a big paper, right? 100 patients. This remains a difficult question: who do you select to do surgery? Three very straightforward variables: lack of small bowel feces sign, obstipation, and mesenteric edema. I still use this. Do you guys use it?

LS

Absolutely.

MD

I noticed it says lack of small bowel feces sign, which I thought was interesting because both in training and in my practice, I have always felt that a small bowel feces sign was a worse prognostic factor because there is stasis in the small bowel and the content is not moving forward, but the paper actually indicates that it is lack of that sign which is indicative of failure. I thought this was counterintuitive to what most people practice or how most people interpret the scans.

LS

I agree, and this is one of the novel aspects of this model, because this is a finding that you frequently see reported as a sign of high-grade bowel obstruction. So, it starts with a CT reading, and it percolates through the various individuals caring for the patient. So, if you have a patient with small bowel obstruction whom you remotely operated on, he/she is likely to be admitted to Hospital Internal Medicine, at least in our practice. Therefore, we may have another team involved in the patient's care who presents the case to us as a serious condition, implying that it could require surgery, whereas when I see myself the small bowel feces sign and no mesenteric edema on the CT, I can feel at least in part reassured even before I examine the patient. However, there are cases that are in a gray area, and so, despite the usefulness of the model, not all the criteria might be met or the findings are contradictory. So, we still have to exert our clinical judgment.

MD

And these remain very difficult cases, but I think that if I see a patient that has a small bowel feces sign, generally, it is a positive, encouraging finding. And then, of course, the edema is something that is more uniform in its interpretation and lack of bowel movements. You can ask this directly to patients, so you don't need to rely on the interpretation of others. And here you have your model. So, I don't use it rigidly, but certainly it helps to decide.

LS

Yes, I agree. Of course, if a patient tells me that they had terrible abdominal pain, they have a heart rate of 120, and they have been fully resuscitated, that will still make a difference. But I think that the existence of a model that has been scientifically tested, and this is just the first paper on it, and then further developed with the use of gastrografin challenge, etc. is very useful. I think it is content you can put directly into practice.

MD

Yeah, I think it's definitely helpful, especially in situations where someone's not progressing as quickly as you'd like. In more of the gray area zones where there is not necessarily hard science data to direct us, I do take the model into account with the addition of the gastrografin challenge. I would usually do it 24 h after the initial

CT scan, depending on the clinical scenario. It's certainly a helpful risk predictive model, I think, with regard to how to manage small bowel obstruction.

DC

Multiple subsequent validation studies later, these variables stuck. Other things were taken into account in subsequent studies like the patient's overall health. But still a valid study. Of course, this may not pan out exactly the same in large bowel obstruction, which is more of what we see, and we need to keep that in mind.

LS

That is a very different scenario, yes.

Reconstructive Surgery After Failed Colorectal Anastomosis

38

Calmels M, Collard MK, O'Connell L, et al. Redo-surgery after failed colorectal or coloanal anastomosis: morbidity, mortality and factors predictive of success. A retrospective study of 200 patients. Colorectal Dis. 2022;24(4):511–9.

Abstract

Aim: In cases of anastomotic failure after colorectal (CRA) or coloanal anastomosis (CAA), revision of the anastomosis is an ambitious surgical option that can be proposed in order to maintain bowel continuity. Our aim was to assess postoperative morbidity, risk of failure, and risk factor for failure in patients after CRA or CAA.

Methods: All consecutive patients who underwent redo-CRA/CAA in our institution between 2007 and 2018 were retrospectively included. The success of redo-CRA/CAA was defined by the restoration of bowel continuity 12 months after the surgery.

Results: Two hundred patients (114 male: 57%) were analyzed. The indication for redo-CRA/CAA was chronic pelvic infection in 74 patients (37%), recto-vaginal or urinary fistula in 59 patients (30%), anastomotic stenosis in 36 patients (18%), and redo anastomosis after previous anastomosis takedown in 31 patients (15%). Twenty-three percent of the patients developed a severe postoperative complication. Anastomotic leakage was diagnosed in 39 patients (20%). One-year-success of the redo-

© The Author(s), under exclusive license to Springer Nature Switzerland AG 2025
D. Colibaseanu et al., *Essential Articles in Colorectal Surgery*,
https://doi.org/10.1007/978-3-031-77745-5_38

CRA/CAA was obtained in 80% of patients. In multivariate analysis, only obesity was associated with redo-CRA/CAA failure ($p = 0.042$). We elaborated a preoperative predictive score of success using the four variables: male sex, age > 60 years, obesity, and history of pelvic radiotherapy. The success of redo-CRA/CAA was 92%, 86%, 80%, and 62% for a preoperative predictive score value of 0, 1, 2 and ≥3, respectively ($p = 0.010$).

Conclusions: In case of failure of primary CRA/CAA, bowel continuity can be saved in 4 out of 5 patients by redo-CRA/CAA despite 23% suffering severe postoperative morbidity.

LS

This article includes a substantial experience of a single unit in the reconstruction of failed colorectal or coloanal anastomoses. The analysis was used to generate a preoperative score predictive of success defined as restoration of intestinal continuity without associated stomas 1 year after redo surgery. The variables used to construct the score included male sex, age >60 years, obesity, and history of pelvic radiotherapy. These are somewhat expected risk factors and with the exception of obesity are not correctable, but the score is practically useful and helpful in patient counseling. The overall success rate of 80%, which varied according to the patient score, is remarkable given the patient population and the recognized risk of permanent stoma creation also associated with index colorectal or colo-anal anastomosis, as the authors also mention in their introduction. Reconstruction after failed low anterior resection is rarely advertised as a surgical service line and might seem like a niche practice, but complications after primary surgery can and do occur, so these are certainly patients whom a colorectal surgeon working in a tertiary referral center could be realistically asked to evaluate. In the assessment of candidates for a reconstructive procedure aimed at functional improvement, rather than preservation of life, patient selection is paramount, as the authors also point out. It is therefore not surprising that the authors considered for reconstruction only patients with an American Society of Anesthesiology classification below 3 with few exceptions. The other important aspect of the patient evaluation for this condition is that reconstructive surgery under these circumstances can be associated with suboptimal functional outcomes, and therefore, an honest and candid discussion is necessary to understand if the patient is really motivated. The 6% secondary stoma creation rate due to poor function after redo anastomosis among patients in the present series confirms the appropriateness of patient selection, although there might have been a number of technically successful cases associated with various degrees of low anterior resection syndrome and/or fecal incontinence. However, for selected, motivated individuals, these long-term complications remain preferable to a permanent stoma. The article also references some fundamental techniques for colonic mobilization to achieve a tension-free redo anastomosis such as the Toupet procedure [1] also known as retroileal anastomosis and Deloyers procedure [2] also known as right colon derotation. Reconstruction of the colorectal or colo-anal anastomosis was carried out using a stapled technique when possible. When this was not possible, alternative advanced techniques of reconstruction included the Soave procedure [3], which is a handsewn coloanal anastomosis after mucosectomy conducted using a combined anterior and perineal approach, and the delayed coloanal anastomosis, also known in the United States as Turnbull-Cutait pull-through [4, 5]. Besides the applicability of the predictive score of 1-year success, this article stands out as a beautiful showcase of those advanced techniques which surgeons should have at their disposal when faced with a difficult colorectal or colo-anal anastomosis construction.

References

1. Toupet A. [Colonectomies with transmesenteric anastomosis]. Mem Acad Chir (Paris). 1963;89:628–30. French.
2. Jouvin I, Pocard M, Najah H. Deloyers procedure. J Visc Surg. 2018;155(6):493–501.
3. Lefèvre JH, Parc Y. Soave procedure. J Visc Surg. 2011;148(4):e262–6.

4. Turnbull RB Jr, Cuthberson A. Abdominorectal pull-through resection for cancer and for Hirschsprung's disease. Delayed posterior colorectal anastomosis. Cleve Clin Q. 1961;28:109–15.
5. Cutait DE, Figliolini FJ. A new method of colorectal anastomosis in abdominoperineal resection. Dis Colon Rectum. 1961;4:335–42.

Discussion

DC

One easy-to-overlook aspect of this article is that the high technical success rate is in patients that were carefully selected as good candidates for salvage surgery. Without taking anything from the excellent outcomes and techniques described, we must remember that it is critical to select appropriate patients for this. Leading into my second point, as the authors astutely point out, technical success is not necessarily functional success. As they point out in another published work, they see that less than half of the patients have an excellent functional outcome. Thirdly, this type of surgery requires a special type of surgeon, not only with experience and excellent skills but also the temperament to guide the patients through a difficult recovery and oftentimes an adjustment to their new physiology.

LS

I agree. Besides its inherent value, I found this article impressive in the way it showcased the practical use of various time-honored surgical techniques to achieve a successful colorectal or coloanal anastomosis. It feels as if this article could be still remarkable just based on its reference list!

AM

I agree, this is a great article that really outlines many of these important surgical techniques. The fundamental aspect of redo-surgery, whether to re-establish intestinal continuity or not, is patient selection and expectation. This includes, as the authors suggest, expectations with regard to the technical success of being liberated from an ostomy and functional success. Technical success is much more easily defined—does the patient have a stoma or not? Functional success is completely dependent upon the patient—are they more satisfied with an improved quality of life than when they had a stoma?

Surgeon vs. Patient Perspectives on Managing Treatment-Associated Risks

39

Solomon MJ, Pager CK, Keshava A, et al. What do patients want? Patient preferences and surrogate decision making in the treatment of colorectal cancer. Dis Colon Rectum. 2003;46(10):1351–7.

Abstract

Purpose: Clinicians often make decisions for their patients, despite evidence that suggests that correspondence between patient and clinician decision making is poor. The management of colorectal cancer presents difficult decisions because the impact of treatment on quality of life might overshadow its survival efficacy. This study investigated whether patients are able to trade survival for quality of life as a means to express their preference for treatment options and to compare their preferences with those expressed by clinicians.

Methods: Patients undergoing curative surgery for colorectal cancer were interviewed postoperatively to elicit their preferences in four hypothetical treatment scenarios. A questionnaire was mailed to all Australian colorectal surgeons and medical oncologists that asked them to respond as if they themselves were patients.

Results: One hundred patients (91%), 43 colorectal surgeons (77%), and 103 medical oncologists (50%) participated. In all four scenarios, patients were able to trade survival for quality of life. Patients' responses varied between scenarios, both in willingness to trade and the average amount traded. There were significant differences between patients and clinicians. Clinicians were more willing than patients to trade survival to avoid a permanent colostomy in favor of chemoradiotherapy. Patients' strongest preference was to avoid chemotherapy, more than to avoid a permanent colostomy.

Conclusions: Patients are able to trade survival as a measure of preference for quality of life and can do so differentially between treatment scenarios. Patients' preferences do not always accord with those of clinicians. Unless patients' preferences are explicitly sought and incorporated into clinical decision-making, patients may not receive the treatment that is best for them.

LS

The difference between doctor and patient perception of priorities in the management of various conditions is an evolving dilemma which relates to our society and culture. It is sometimes assumed that the treating doctor should be the most effective patient advocate since he/she is at once intimately knowledgeable of the patient's condition but also presumably close to the patient as a person with their individual circumstances. However, this is only true to a certain extent, and the patient may well have different views on treatments and should express and ultimately receive their preferred treatment option, provided it is medically sound. This was a study focused on cancer where the data were collected through questionnaires mailed not only to patients, but also to medical oncologists and surgeons, asking them to respond when imagining themselves being the patients. Four different scenarios were presented, and in one which is quite familiar to many colorectal surgeons, patients were willing to trade survival time in exchange for avoidance of colostomy through local excision of rectal cancer. This is a study conducted in Australia in the early 2000s. It was the first piece of evidence that I read investigating these issues, and it is important because it underscores the differences in perspective between doctors and patients. The specific questions and answers might seem at times obsolete or irrelevant in this day and age in the United States. For example, it was surprising to see that the patients included in this study indicated their preference for surgical resection and colostomy to avoid chemotherapy. Given the widespread success of nonoperative management of rectal cancer, this is the opposite of what we would typically expect today. A particularly challenging situation is when a patient asks for a treatment which the surgeon would not recommend. In this case, one option is to decline treating the patient altogether and refer him/her for another opinion. Another approach is to accept some compromise based on the principle that some treatment is better than no treatment. These conversations poorly lend themselves to a one-size-fits-all approach and should be managed based on their individual circumstances. A more recent systematic review of 37 studies once more underscored differences between physician and patient preferences in a variety of cancer treatments [1]. In general, patients are more willing to accept the increased risk associated with treatments in exchange for potential health benefits and better quality of life when compared to clinicians, who emphasize more the adverse effects associated with treatments. In another older study on the management of dysplasia in the background of ulcerative colitis, 60% of patients responded in a survey that they would refuse a physician's recommendation for elective colectomy if dysplasia were detected despite being told that they had a 20% risk of having cancer at the time of their conversation [2]. The management of dysplasia in the background of ulcerative colitis has changed since 2007 when the study was conducted, and many of the patients who were offered surgery at that time would be treated with endoscopic excision today. However, this study in inflammatory bowel disease confirms the findings of the cancer studies mentioned above in that it points out how frequently patients are willing to trade some risk of their own lives in exchange for what they value as an important quality-of-life benefit. As caregivers, our obligation is to provide sound medical information to patients and allow them an informed decision. This is a principle which should inform our daily practice regardless of how difficult its implementation is.

References

1. Zhang M, He X, Wu J, Xie F. Differences between physician and patient preferences for cancer treatments: a systematic review. BMC Cancer. 2023;23(1):1126.
2. Siegel CA, Schwartz LM, Woloshin S, et al. When should ulcerative colitis patients undergo colectomy for dysplasia? Mismatch between patient preferences and physician recommendations. Inflamm Bowel Dis. 2010;16(10):1658–62.

Discussion

DC

This was published in 2002. It was the avant-garde of many studies that have since been published on this pretty complex topic to study. And so, what it found was very interesting because it brought to light what probably many suspected, which is that the preferences of the patients are not always the same as the providers. They have different priorities sometimes and a different understanding and obviously a different experience of what is happening to them.

MD

As clinicians, particularly as cancer surgeons, our primary concern typically revolves around ensuring patient survival. This overarching principle guides our recommendations when caring for individuals with cancer. Within our specialty, where procedures like colostomies and ileostomies may be necessary, even with the potential for restoration of intestinal continuity, significant alterations in bowel function can profoundly impact the quality of life. Therefore, I find papers such as this one particularly pertinent to our practice. What intrigued me most was the disparity between the approaches of surgeons and oncologists in weighing survival against the risks and benefits of surgical procedures versus chemotherapy. Notably, in this study, patients expressed a preference for a colostomy over chemotherapy, a sentiment that may have shifted over time, especially with the growing acceptance of watch-and-wait strategies for rectal cancer.

In addition, I make a concerted effort to prioritize patients' well-being, taking into account factors such as their quality of life, baseline health, and preferences. However, there are instances, such as those discussed at tumor board meetings, where patient preferences may conflict with our medical recommendations. For example, when a patient desires a transanal excision for a T2N0 lesion with lymphovascular invasion, despite our reservations due to its potential impact on survival, it becomes a challenging decision. While we may feel uneasy offering procedures associated with decreased survival rates over alternatives that could significantly enhance the quality of life, it underscores the complex interplay between patient preference and medical judgment highlighted in this paper.

DC

Do you guys get the impression that patients were pretty freaked out about chemotherapy?

LS

This particular finding of the Solomon paper was also surprising to me, and honestly, it does not seem to correlate with what I see in practice, particularly in the area of watch and wait as Michelle pointed out.

This is probably the first original paper that I read which confronted me in a scientific way with the experience that I developed when facing clinical scenarios and giving recommendations. And I share the same view as Michelle in that survival and cure from cancer are the preeminent goals. I have tried to put myself in a patient's shoes. If I were the patient and I were that very person who could avoid a colostomy and take some risk of death, I think that it is conceivable that I could decide to do that. I have come to respect it, and still, it is difficult to navigate the intricacies of where you draw the line between where you say "this is not really what I recommend, but I still do it for the patient" vs. "there are certain things that the patient is asking that I'm not in agreement with, and the patient will need to find another surgeon." Because of experiences like the ones reported here, I feel I have a more nuanced approach and respect for the patient's personal preference as one of the stakeholders, so I do not feel offended by engaging in a sort of health bargaining. But at the same time, I do need to draw lines in certain areas. And I have to tell patients, for example, if you do TNT for rectal cancer and, after all the radiotherapy and chemotherapy, you have regrowth in the anal sphincter, I need to tell patients that they need an APR. And I cannot accept that the patient says, well, let us continue with some more chemotherapy; apart from that, the oncologist would probably not be in agreement with this approach. I need to tell this patient that this is not what I recommend. I recommend surgery, and in this case, it would unfortunately involve a colostomy creation.

MD

I think that.

LS

There is this expression that I learned from our colleague Amit Merchea when a patient asks for a lesser procedure rather than a radical procedure recommended by a surgeon. Amit feels that in many of those situations we should "at least do something." For example, the patient wants a local excision. You would not really do a local excision, but you accept to do it because at least you do something for the patient.

DC

I think the first step in doing something is learning where the patient is coming from and making sure that—best I can—I do a good job of educating the patient.

MD

And rightly so, but I think it is still so much upon us to ultimately decide.

Comparison of Surgical Treatments for Rectal Prolapse

40

Senapati A, Gray RG, Middleton LJ, et al. PROSPER: a randomised comparison of surgical treatments for rectal prolapse. Colorectal Dis. 2013;15(7):858–68.

Abstract

Aim: Rectal prolapse is a profoundly disabling condition, occurring mainly in elderly and parous women. There is no accepted standard surgical treatment, with previous studies limited in methodological quality and size. PROSPER aimed to address these deficiencies by comparing the relative merits of different procedures.

Method: In a pragmatic, factorial (2 × 2) design trial, patients could be randomized between abdominal and perineal surgery (i), and suture versus resection rectopexy for those receiving an abdominal procedure (ii) or Altemeier's versus Delorme's for those receiving a perineal procedure (iii). Primary outcome measures were recurrence of the prolapse, incontinence, bowel function, and quality of life scores (Vaizey, bowel thermometer and EQ-5D) measured up to 3 years.

Results: Two hundred and ninety-three patients were recruited: 49 were randomized between surgical approaches (i); 78 between abdominal procedures (ii); and 213 between perineal procedures (iii). Recurrence rates were higher than anticipated, but not significantly different in any comparison: Altemeier's versus Delorme's

© The Author(s), under exclusive license to Springer Nature Switzerland AG 2025

D. Colibaseanu et al., *Essential Articles in Colorectal Surgery*, https://doi.org/10.1007/978-3-031-77745-5_40

24/102 (24%) and 31/99 (31%) [hazard ratio (HR) 0.81; 95% CI 0.47, 1.38; $P = 0.4$]; resection versus suture rectopexy 4/32 (13%) and 9/35 (26%) (HR 0.45; 95% CI 0.14, 1.46; $P = 0.2$); perineal versus abdominal 5/25 (20%) and 5/19 (26%) (HR 0.83; 95% CI 0.24, 2.86; $P = 0.8$). Vaizey, bowel thermometer, and EQ-5D scores were not significantly different in any of the comparisons.

Conclusion: No significant differences were seen in any of the randomized comparisons, although substantial improvements from baseline in quality of life were noted following all procedures.

LS

The PROSPER (PROlapse Surgery PErineal or Rectopexy) study assessed four different procedures for treatment of rectal prolapse and compared respective rates of prolapse recurrence, fecal incontinence, bowel function, and quality-of-life scores measured up to 3 years postoperatively. Through a complex factorial (2 × 2) design, patients were initially randomized between abdominal and perineal procedures. Subsequent randomization between suture rectopexy versus resection rectopexy occurred within the abdominal treatment arm. If the patient had been initially randomized to the perineal treatment arm, a further randomization occurred between Altemeier procedure and Delorme's procedure. The surgeon could elect to participate in either one or both of the randomization steps, but only randomized patients were ultimately analyzed. This multicenter trial recruited patients from 34 different centers, 30 of which were in the United Kingdom. However, recruitment took over 7 years, and the original target of 950 patients was reduced to 300. Despite this limitation, PROSPER remains the largest trial on surgical treatment of rectal prolapse to date. Probably, the most remarkable and sobering finding is the relatively high recurrence rate after any of the procedures performed. When assessing all patients including those that had not been randomized, the recurrence rate after abdominal procedures was 19%, and the recurrence after perineal procedures was 28%. However, patients undergoing surgery experienced significant postoperative improvements in their bowel function and quality of life. These favorable changes were also not significantly different depending on the specific surgical procedure performed.

The subsequent Swedish rectal prolapse trial shared similar difficulties in patient accrual and showed similar results after a median follow-up of 2.6 years both in terms of improved bowel function scores and high prolapse recurrence rates, which were not significantly different when comparing different surgical procedures. At least 20 percent of the recurrences occurred later than 3 years after surgery [1]. One of the limitations of both the PROSPER and the Swedish rectal prolapse trial is that anterior rectopexy was not among the procedures analyzed. This is a more recently introduced technique which especially when using minimally invasive approaches could be associated with improvement in functional results and reduced rates of prolapse recurrence when compared to the abdominal and perineal procedures analyzed in those trials. The NORDIC rectal prolapse study will evaluate laparoscopic ventral mesh rectopexy as the preferred operation which will be compared in a noninferiority study design to other well-established procedures for rectal prolapse [2]. A network meta-analysis based on nine randomized controlled trials indicated that posterior mesh rectopexy had significantly lower odds of recurrence than did the Altemeier procedure, Delorme procedure, resection rectopexy, sponge rectopexy, and sutured rectopexy, but similar odds to ventral mesh rectopexy [3]. At this time, there is no statistically significant data from individual randomized trials indicating a specific surgical procedure which should be viewed as the most preferable standard of care. In the absence of definitive scientific data, most surgeons probably agree that an abdominal repair is associated with a decreased risk of prolapse recurrence when compared to a perineal approach, which should be generally reserved for high-risk patients.

References

1. Smedberg J, Graf W, Pekkari K, Hjern F. Comparison of four surgical approaches for rectal prolapse: multicentre randomized clinical trial. BJS Open. 2022;6(1):zrab140. https://doi.org/10.1093/bjsopen/zrab140.
2. Bach-Nielsen A, Christensen P, Cornish J, et al. The NORDIC rectal prolapse study: a multicenter international cohort study. Colorectal Dis. 2023;25(S2):239–40.

3. Emile SH, Khan SM, Garoufalia Z, et al. A network meta-analysis of surgical treatments of complete rectal prolapse. Tech Coloproctol. 2023;27(10):787–97.

Discussion

DC

They make the point that this was the largest trial at the time, in 2013, and indeed, finding 293 surgical patients with rectal prolapse is no small feat. I think the intention was good. It was hard (and in some ways, it still is) to know what to do with a patient with rectal prolapse when all nonoperative measures have failed or they are not a candidate for nonoperative measures. Which surgery is best, and in what patient? I think this was the general question they were looking at in a general sense. Definitely, the trial design was the Achilles heel of this study. Yes, 293 patients entered the study, but Fig. 2 is very telling; on one hand, the procedure (abdominal vs perineal) was randomized in 49 patients, and on another, the decision to randomize was made after the decision was already made to proceed abdominally or perineally, where the perineal approach was much more likely to be favored (2.7 times more likely). So ultimately there was randomization, but the way it was done and also the small (and multiple) group sizes made it tough to detect a difference if there would have been one. As an aside, I think that the perineal group is probably too big, and it is likely that more people than strictly necessary are having the Altemeier procedure, knowing that the recurrence rate is higher than with an abdominal approach.

MD

I think it sounds like the Delorme procedure is much more popular in the UK because it seemed that they do more of that rather than Altemeier. I was very surprised to see that there was no difference between Delorme and Altemeier procedures with regard to recurrence because anecdotally, and I think in other studies, perhaps where there is less experience with the Delorme procedure, the recurrence is usually higher with the Delorme. I was also very surprised to see that they did not show any difference between abdominal versus perineal procedures with regard to recurrence because other studies or meta-analyses looking at a conglomerate of randomized trials have shown more so that recurrence is less with abdominal operations. I think in this trial the original plan was to recruit 900 patients, and 300 is quite commendable, but I do not think that the study is necessarily powered enough to find the differences that they initially were looking for. And the other thing was that they talked about bowel function using the score between patients, but not of other things that affect the recurrence of prolapse, like concomitant vaginal prolapse, the degree of the prolapse, etc., factors which I think significantly affect recurrence for these patients. And the last thing that has been gaining more traction now is ventral mesh rectopexy and whether or not that is a better repair than a posterior approach. Another aspect is not having robotic surgery. I think that now with robotic surgery, the dissection can be visualized more clearly, and perhaps, a more distal dissection is facilitated. Whether or not that makes a difference with regard to abdominal operations, I think, is still unknown, but overall, I think this was a large study for a patient population that is, in general, hard to study and hard to recruit.

LS

I think that if you look at all the abdominal procedures combined vs. all the perineal procedures combined, there is a difference, but it does not reach statistical significance. And I do believe that it is because the study is underpowered to detect that. Some patients have complex pelvic floor prolapse to be repaired at the same time especially in centers specialized in pelvic floor disease, which might require a perineal repair, as Michelle was alluding to. Personally, I try very hard to do an abdominal repair unless there are specific circumstances. For example, the prolapse is short or in case of an urgent operation for ischemic rectal prolapse. I try to avoid a perineal procedure as much as possible. And I think that the bar has shifted in terms of the definition of high risk, and there are a lot of patients who used to be defined as high risk who are actually capable of tolerating an abdominal procedure and therefore achieving the advantages of a reduced recurrence rate. In addition, I would offer resection rectopexy, which is one of the procedures included in the randomization, only in case of prolapse associated with constipation, which I rarely see. Perhaps, with the advent of ventral rectopexy, which has been proposed also for rectal prolapse associated with constipation, this will become even less common.

I commend the investigators of this trial, and I noted that the subsequent Swedish rectal prolapse trial was similar and was faced with the same patient accrual challenges. PROSPER's factorial design did not help in obtaining a result which was statistically significant. But this is the best science that we have, and hopefully, newer trials will incorporate ventral rectopexy so that we can have more definitive results.

Publisher Correction to: Essential Articles in Colorectal Surgery

Publisher Correction to:
D. Colibaseanu et al.,
Essential Articles in Colorectal Surgery,
https://doi.org/10.1007/978-3-031-77745-5

This book was inadvertently published with an incorrect TOC level. We have updated the TOC level.

The updated version of this book can be found at
https://doi.org/10.1007/978-3-031-77745-5

© The Author(s), under exclusive license to Springer Nature
Switzerland AG 2025
D. Colibaseanu et al., *Essential Articles in Colorectal Surgery*,
https://doi.org/10.1007/978-3-031-77745-5_41

Index

© The Editor(s) (if applicable) and The Author(s), under exclusive   291
license to Springer Nature Switzerland AG 2025
D. Colibaseanu et al., *Essential Articles in Colorectal Surgery*,
https://doi.org/10.1007/978-3-031-77745-5

GPSR Compliance

*The European Union's (EU) General Product Safety Regulation (GPSR)
is a set of rules that requires consumer products to be safe and our
obligations to ensure this.*

*If you have any concerns about our products, you can contact us on
ProductSafety@springernature.com*

In case Publisher is established outside the EU, the EU authorized
representative is:

Springer Nature Customer Service Center GmbH
Europaplatz 3
69115 Heidelberg, Germany

Batch number: 10091875

Printed by Printforce, the Netherlands